THRIVE WITH ADULT ADHD WORKBOOK FOR WOMEN

Effective Exercises & Strategies to Improve Focus and Motivation, Executive Functioning. Living Confidently for Women With ADHD

Kai M. Jordan

Swenett Publishing

To you,
To the Mother,
To the sister,
To the daughter,
To the wife,
To the grandmother,

I can't imagine life without you...

CONTENTS

INTRODUCTION

Did you know that women with ADHD (Attention Deficit/Hyperactivity Disorder) are often misdiagnosed and misunderstood, leaving them struggling with untreated symptoms for years and sometimes even decades? This workbook is here to help you break free from the shackles of your diagnosis and unlock your true potential.

This workbook is designed to help women with ADHD understand their condition and develop effective management strategies. It provides a comprehensive guide to ADHD, including its symptoms, causes, and common co-occurring conditions.

Through a series of practical exercises and activities, this workbook offers women with ADHD the tools they need to better understand themselves and their situation. It is a guide to understanding the condition and a tool for building resilience, confidence, and self-acceptance. Whether you have just been diagnosed with ADHD or have been managing the state for years, this workbook is here to help you on your journey to success and fulfillment.

Before diving into the book, check out a few common ADHD difficulties:

- Do you find it difficult to concentrate, and are you easily distracted?
- Do you need help to start or finish projects?
- Do you often experience mood swings, feel restless, or have trouble relaxing?
- Do you need help with time management or staying on schedule?
- Do you need help staying quiet and frequently interrupting others?
- Do you find it challenging to make your point when speaking?
- Do you tend to start new projects before completing old ones?
- Do you have an affinity to indulge in dangerous activities with little or no regard for safety?

If your answer is "yes" to most of these questions, you might be an adult with ADHD; if that is the case, there's a lot you can do to improve your life.

As an author and advocate for women with ADHD, I am thrilled to be creating a workbook on this topic. My passion for this subject stem from a deep desire to help women with ADHD feel validated, understood, and empowered. I believe that women with ADHD are a unique and underserved population, often struggling in silence and feeling like they don't quite fit in.

However, ADHD can also come with many strengths and gifts, such as creativity, empathy, and a unique perspective on the world. By focusing on these strengths while providing practical tools and strategies for managing ADHD symptoms, I hope to help women with ADHD build their confidence and achieve their goals. This workbook is a labor of love, and I am committed to providing the best possible resource for women with ADHD. I believe that with the proper knowledge and support, women with ADHD can overcome their challenges, embrace their strengths, and live a fulfilling and successful life.

If you're reading this workbook, chances are you've experienced the frustration of being told to "just focus" or "just get organized." I want you to know that I understand the unique challenges of ADHD and validate your experiences. You are not alone, and I'm here to help you navigate the ups and downs of life with ADHD. I believe that women with ADHD have so much potential, and I can't wait to help them discover their strengths and reach their goals. Let's dive in and explore the world of ADHD together!

◆ ◆ ◆

YOUR FREE GIFT

As a way of saying thanks for your purchase, I'm offering ***The ADHD Relationship Evaluation and Money Management Worksheet*** for FREE to my readers.

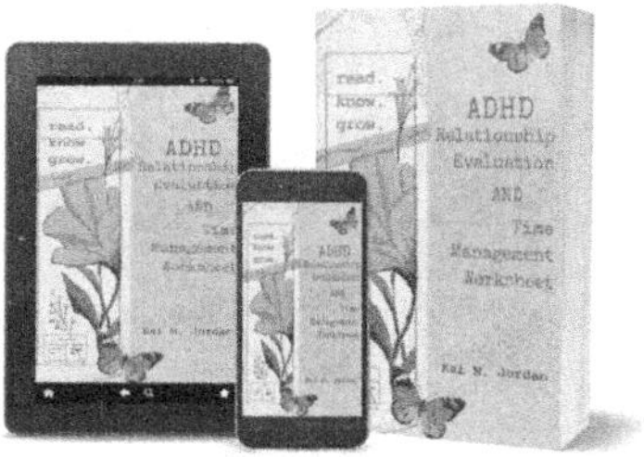

Plus, you will also get my ***Declutter Your Mind Bundle*** for FREE, which includes four valuable components:

1. Loving Yourself EXECUTIVE SUMMARY (Action Guide)

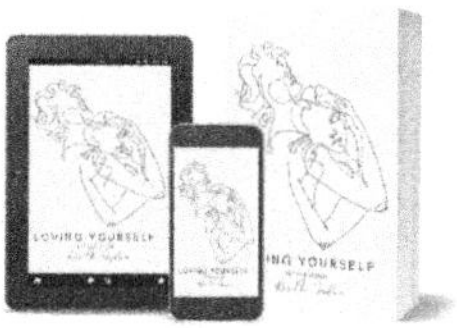

2. Daily Routines to Tackle Your Biggest Worry (Action Guide)

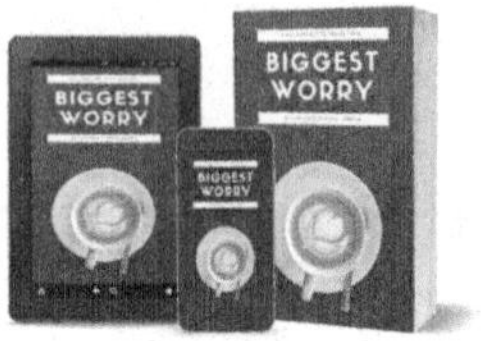

3. Decluttering Your Mind Worksheet

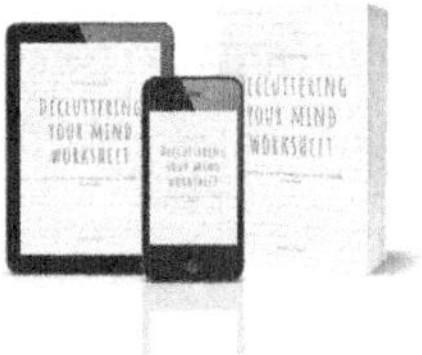

4. Decluttering Your Mind Checklist

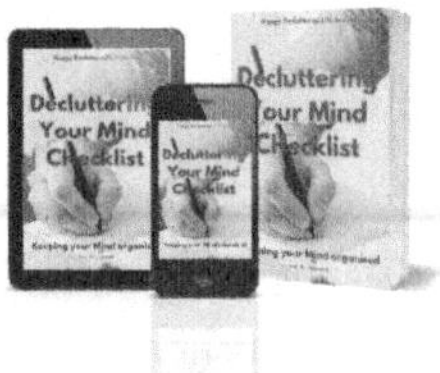

To get access to your FREE bonuses, just go to:

http://swenettbooks.com

or Just Scan this Code by Your Phone

If you want to get the maximum benefit through your reading journey, make sure to grab the free bundle NOW!

This book belongs to

ABOUT THE AUTHOR

Kai M. Jordan is an Amazon best-selling author in self-development, home management, and lifestyle coaching. Visit http://swenettbooks.com and get access to Kai's bonuses for FREE.

In her books, Kai shares over ten years of practical knowledge and the timeless wisdom she learned from an early age about managing homes, mind, and life by self-discovery and self-management. She turns these life lessons into actionable steps to help you develop a healthy relationship with yourself, others, and life itself.

In her honest and inspiring books, Kai talks about what she believes are the obstacles to living your desired life. She shares best practices to help you declutter your mind, home & life, deal with your ADHD, improve powerful habits, erase negativity, control anxiety, reduce overthinking, and minimize any expectations of others. She guides YOU to think, decide and become the best version of yourself.

Kai studied business administration and management. When she's not on her mission to improve people's lives, she loves to read, meditate, work out, and take long walks in nature.

◆ ◆ ◆

HOW TO USE THIS BOOK?

If you're a woman with ADHD, you know that managing your symptoms can be challenging.

This ADHD workbook is designed specifically for women.

It can be a helpful resource for developing new skills and strategies to manage your symptoms and address the unique challenges of being a woman with ADHD. It's not just an ordinary theoretical book; ***it's loaded with practical exercises*** and advice you can apply *daily.* This is what makes this book special.

Start by reading through the introduction and other relevant sections that provide an overview of the book and its purpose. It will give you a sense of the workbook's intended audience and goals.

Take note of specific issues or challenges unique

to women with ADHD. This workbook for women covers topics such as hormonal changes, managing relationships, or balancing work and family responsibilities.

- **Identify your areas of interest or concern**. Consider which areas you would like to focus on, and prioritize accordingly. This workbook covers various topics, such as self-esteem, anxiety, and emotional regulation.

- **Set realistic goals for yourself.** Break the workbook into manageable chunks and make sure each goal is achievable. It's essential to be honest about what you can realistically accomplish within a given timeframe.

- **Take as many breaks as needed.** ADHD workbooks can be time-consuming and challenging, so taking breaks as needed is essential. Use this time to engage in activities that help you relax and recharge.

- **Try to stay organized**. Ensure you have a system for organizing your thoughts and tracking your progress. Depending on the format of the workbook, you may need to keep track of your responses or notes in a separate notebook or journal.

- **Be open to learning and growth.** The purpose

of this ADHD workbook is to help you develop new skills and strategies for managing your symptoms and addressing issues unique to women. Approach each exercise with an open mind and a willingness to learn and grow.

- **Consider seeking additional support.** While this ADHD workbook can be a helpful resource, it's essential to work with a healthcare professional who understands the unique challenges of ADHD in women. Consider seeking additional support from a therapist, coach, or support group to help you implement the strategies and skills you learn from the workbook.

In short, this workbook helps manage your symptoms and address the unique challenges of being a woman with ADHD.

Following the instructions can get the most out of your workbook and develop new skills and strategies for managing your symptoms. Boost your confidence and design your personalized plan using the exercises and tips in the book.

◆ ◆ ◆

CHAPTER 1: ADHD...WHAT IS IT? HOW DOES IT AFFECT ME?

ADHD is not something you outgrow; it's something you learn to manage. –Dr. Russell Barkley

Imagine watching your favorite movie on a TV with a poor signal. The picture keeps flickering, the sound is distorted, and you can't seem to focus on what's happening. That's what it can feel like to have ADHD. This chapter will explore what this disorder is and how it affects you.

You'll discover the science behind ADHD and better understand how it impacts your daily life. By the end of this chapter, you'll be better equipped to recognize your unique challenges and strengths and ready to start taking control of your ADHD.

In this chapter, we'll cover everything from identifying symptoms of ADHD and how they can impact your daily life to exploring a personalized treatment plan that works for you. We'll also dive into the importance of setting achievable goals and how to use your ADHD strengths to your advantage.

Attention Deficit/Hyperactivity Disorder is a precise, scientifically acknowledged term that applies to all types of this disorder (for example, ADHD-inattentive, ADHD-hyperactive, or ADHD-combined subtypes). The ideas and exercises in this book will help you design unique approaches and make the most of available resources and professional assistance.

Have you ever struggled with concentration, interrupted people while they were talking, had difficulty sitting quietly, or behaved impulsively despite the possibility of danger? Most people, including children and adults, occasionally encounter these difficulties, but those with ADHD may experience them daily.

Your functioning will be impacted by ADHD symptoms which may lead you to think, "Can

I grow out of it? Can things get any worse? What therapies are most effective for me?" These questions are common and reasonable. With the correct information, you can discover precisely what ADHD is and how to manage its symptoms.

This particular disorder is a common neurodevelopmental condition that impacts behavior. Inability to focus, impulsivity, hyperactivity, and chronic patterns of inattention are common symptoms.

These tendencies might make it difficult for you to function normally and learn new skills. However, not everyone with this diagnosis has the same symptoms. ADHD is often identified in children between 6 and 12, although symptoms can appear at any age. Suppose you were diagnosed with ADHD later in life. In that case, it might signify that you had symptoms from childhood, but they went unnoticed or were misdiagnosed.

In women, ADHD can often present differently than in men, leading to underdiagnosis or misdiagnosis. Women with ADHD may be less likely to exhibit hyperactivity symptoms and more likely to experience inattentiveness and impulsivity. This can lead to difficulties in academic or work settings and difficulty maintaining social relationships. Women with ADHD may also experience anxiety, depression, and low self-esteem due to their symptoms.

ADHD is classified into three categories:

- **Inattentive ADHD**: People with this type of ADHD struggle to pay attention, stay organized, and complete tasks. They may appear forgetful, disorganized, and easily distracted.

- **Hyperactive-impulsive ADHD:** People with this type may be very active, fidgety, and restless. They may also struggle with impulsivity, acting without thinking through consequences, interrupting others, and having difficulty waiting their turn.

- **Combined ADHD:** People with this type of ADHD have both inattentive and hyperactivity/impulsivity symptoms. They may struggle with paying attention, completing tasks, staying organized, and being restless, fidgety, and impulsive.

It's important to note that ADHD symptoms can vary significantly from person to person, and not everyone will exhibit all symptoms associated with a particular type. Consulting a medical professional for an accurate diagnosis and appropriate treatment is essential.

Realize Your Symptoms

While some women with ADHD are restless and energetic, others are far more inactive and find it challenging to get started. Some women can't resist scrolling through social media while there is an impending deadline; others perform better under pressure yet struggle to fill out the necessary paperwork.

When going through the following characteristics to determine whether they fit your experience, consider them in the setting of a regular day rather than any exciting situation when you're pumped up with adrenaline. When someone is engaged in activities that don't appear extremely interesting, ADHD symptoms become considerably more apparent.

◆ ◆ ◆

Date -------

Exercise 1

Make a note of which of these characteristics influences your daily life so you can consider them as we move further in this book:

- **Forgetful:** In many ways, forgetfulness impacts life, including leaving your things behind at home, forgetting to make an important phone call, and ignoring essential emails.

- **Underachiever:** ADHD shows up as underachievement in adults. Since they cannot perform at a level consistent with their IQ, many people with ADHD struggle. They may have a history of problems in their jobs or relationships.

- **Stagnant:** Feeling stuck is a life pattern for people with ADHD. The energy required to excel in school, work, or to accomplish other goals is depleted by ADHD traits. This feeling of being trapped causes persistent hopelessness about the future.

- **Time blindness:** Many people with ADHD misjudge how long tasks will take. When they are engaged in an activity that stimulates them, they lose track of time, which causes them to be late and rush through tasks constantly. They usually don't know how much should be done in a day; therefore, they're never sure if they have accomplished enough.

- **Slacker**: Most people put off paying bills, returning phone calls, or going to the gym. However, for some people with ADHD, the tasks keep piling up because getting started on specific tasks is challenging and seems almost impossible.

- **Impulsive**: Impulsivity comes in many forms. It involves verbal impulsivity, interrupting others in conversation, spending money carelessly, frequently changing your mind, acting without thinking through the repercussions, and starting or leaving a job without research. Even a little impulsivity can have severe repercussions in an adult's life. It could manifest as reckless driving or binging on food, drink, or drugs.

- **Novelty seeking:** The characteristic of novelty seeking is the desire for the new. The mind cannot control boredom and is always drawn to the next exciting thing. This might make it quite challenging to finish tasks. There are too many obligations to meet. Even maintaining a relationship can be difficult because of what people do to avoid boredom—oversleeping, overeating, playing video games for hours, and immersing themselves in social media rather than doing their work. Some people use their craving for novelty and lack of self-control as a gateway to drugs, alcohol, or other harmful habits.

- **Distractible**: Of all the ADHD symptoms, distractibility may be the most common one. Many women with ADHD have focus issues. They could devote hours of attention to a topic of interest yet struggle to pay attention to other aspects of life. They can have too many thoughts running through their minds simultaneously, making concentrating on just one complex. It might be impossible to study or work in a crowded place.

- **Disorganized**: Not all women with ADHD are sloppy. Their homes and vehicles may be cluttered. Unorganized women complete work at the last minute, if at all. Moreover, their brains constantly move, making it difficult to complete tasks and converse.

Build My Unique Treatment Plan

The challenge for most women with ADHD is not a lack of ambition or motivation. Instead, ADHD interferes with following through the step-by-step process over time to accomplish those goals, especially when the result is not immediate. For example, everyone wants to be in better physical shape. Still, it can be challenging to stick to a healthier diet and exercise until the desired effects appear.

ADHD can be treated, and its symptoms can be controlled, regardless of when you were first diagnosed. You don't simply grow out of ADHD. In most cases, it calls for the assistance of a medical specialist. Medication, psychotherapy, and behaviour management are common treatments for ADHD. In many cases, a combination of all three is required. Suppose you have ADHD or any mental health disorder.

In that case, starting by treating the symptoms that significantly impact you is best. The treatment of ADHD includes a wide range of prescription drugs. A doctor, psychiatrist, or pediatrician will frequently experiment with several medications and doses to determine the most effective for you and your symptoms. Sometimes the procedure takes a while.

It is considerably more difficult for women with ADHD to break down big tasks into step-by-step strategies and consistently execute these plans. It is crucial to create detailed programs for each part of your day, which help establish the framework and routine of your day.

It is essential if you still need the structure offered by work or school on those days. You may be self-employed, a graduate student, or a stay-at-home mom, all of which require you to create your schedule.

Knowing that you could have ADHD is comfort itself. You can stop criticizing yourself for being unable to shrug off your problems once you realize what's wrong. But without that diagnosis, you can't tell if you have ADHD. Only an experienced mental health specialist has the knowledge and expertise to use the treatment guidelines.

There are multiple steps in a professional evaluation. These procedures are intended to examine your problems from different angles, ensuring that vital information is received and symptoms are understood. The process may appear repetitive to you.

However, remember that the practitioner is attempting to identify all potential causes of your problems and will also gather important details about your unique abilities. You may choose coping mechanisms specifically designed to help you the most by being aware of your strengths in terms of life skills and personal qualities. You may learn to use your creative abilities and engaging personality to compensate for ADHD symptoms.

Finding out precisely what is wrong is the goal of the evaluation process so that a treatment plan may be created to get you on the path to success and health as soon as possible.
A diagnosis of ADHD is like a gateway to a better life. You have access to the following:

- Medication will improve your ability to focus, adapt, manage your time, and fight off distractions.
- Strategies can be used to highlight your strengths.
- Tools can be used to make up for your shortcomings.
- Coping techniques will enhance your productivity in the workplace or the family.
- Support from people who care about your aspirations and your success.

◆ ◆ ◆

Date -------

Exercise 2

Answer the list of trait-based questions that follows. You can use the answers to understand yourself better and collaborate with professionals or therapists. It will make things more transparent and prepare you for the treatment ahead.

Forgetful:

- Do you often need to remember what people have told you?

✓ ....

✕ ....

- Do you need help remembering where you kept things?

✓ ....

✕ ....

- Do you require reminders for routine tasks?

✓ ....

✕ ....

- Do you frequently need to remember about appointments?

✓ ....
✕ ....

Underachiever:

- Do you believe you are performing below your potential in life?

✓ ....
✕ ....

- Should you have gotten better school marks or progressed in your career?

✓ ....
✕ ....

Stagnant:

- Do you find it difficult to advance in life?

✓ ....
✕ ....

- Do you feel stuck in life?

✓ ....
✕ ....

- Do you feel trapped in essential aspects of your life, such as work or school?

✓ ....

✕ ....

Time blindness:

- Do you frequently show up late?

✓ ....

✕ ....

- Do you underestimate how much time things take?

✓ ....

✕ ....

- Does time pass quickly?

✓ ....

✕ ....

Slacker:

- Do you procrastinate?

✓ ....

✕ ....

- Do you require a deadline to motivate you to complete tasks?

✓ ....

✕ ....

- Do you find it challenging to begin lessons?

✓ ....

✕ ....

- Do you often start projects but struggle to finish them?

✓ ....

✕ ....

Impulsive:

- Do you often make decisions without considering the repercussions?

✓ ....

✕ ....

- Do you say things out of turn in conversation?

✓ ....

✕ ....

- Do you make purchases without taking the price or your budget into account?

✓ ....

✗ ....

Novelty seeking:

- Do you get bored quickly?

✓ ....

✗ ....

- Do you try to avoid boredom by seeking out new, exciting experiences?

✓ ....

✗ ....

- Do you say "yes" to more commitments when you're too busy?

✓ ....

✗ ....

Distractible:

- Do sights, noises, thoughts, or less critical tasks cause you to become distracted from what you should be doing?

✓ ....

✗ ....

- Do you frequently catch yourself daydreaming?

✓ ....

✕ ....

Disorganized:

- Do you have a cluttered personal space?

✓ ....

✕ ....

- Do your desk, home, or car appear to be in disarray?

✓ ....

✕ ....

- Do you forget what you have to do and when you have to do it?

✓ ....

✕ ....

When you receive a new diagnosis and learn about all your potential treatment options, it's natural to feel overwhelmed. However, ADHD can be managed, and you can actively participate in this process. You can try several other things to help you cope, as well as medication and psychotherapy, like having a healthy lifestyle.

ADHD and Goals

With ADHD, setting goals might seem impossible. Prioritizing, breaking down work, and setting deadlines can be difficult for a woman with this disorder. The difficulty in estimating time, starting tedious activities, planning, and prioritizing are examples of executive functioning problems.

These are all essential aspects of goal-setting, which might be more difficult for those with ADHD. The relationship between task and reward may also seem different in neurodiverse women compared to neurotypical women. As a result, it is more challenging to create goals and incentives in a way that supports the reward mechanisms of ADHD.

The optimal goal-setting strategy for women with ADHD often considers these difficulties with executive functioning. For example, starting a project might be more challenging if you are motivationally challenged. If working memory is an issue, goals must be written down as part of the process.

It's important to constantly revisit your plans to stay motivated and tackle any obstacles to accomplish them. To focus on how to deal with your executive functioning issues and achieve your goals without getting overwhelmed, remain in a setting where you feel comfortable exploring, experimenting, and resolving.

Strategies to accomplish a plan may change, but if you stay focused on your ultimate goal and understand how stress hormones and challenges may contribute, you can adapt how you accomplish the goal without losing interest.

When discussing goals with ADHD, the focus is on the "what" and "how" a plan would be accomplished. The acronym SMART is one method to understand the "how" and "what." SMART stands for specific, measurable, achievable, relevant, and time-based. Any goals set should ideally discuss these components. For example, a plan to "be more productive" is an example that doesn't fit the SMART requirements. For that goal to be more precise regarding both the "what" and "how," it must be:

- **Specific**: Concentrate on accomplishing tedious tasks at hand. Instead of trying to become a great artist, the goal should be to sketch for at least an hour every day. It answers questions like, "What do you want to achieve, and how will you do it?"

- **Measured**: Concentrate on a single activity for a considerable amount of time.

Instead of saying you want to learn to play an instrument, make a goal to spend an hour practicing every day. Use numbers in your plan.

- **Achievable**: Focus on existing rather than upcoming tasks. It might be unrealistic to set a goal of becoming a doctor if you hate biology. Your goal must be something you can accomplish.

- **Relevant**: Why is your goal important to you? It will be far more challenging to fulfill your dream of exercising three days a week if you're doing it only because you've heard it's healthy for you rather than because it makes you feel good.
- **Time-based**: Set deadlines for your goal and any necessary subgoals. This may change later, but measuring your progress without a deadline is far more complicated.

◆ ◆ ◆

Date ---------

Exercise 3

Having ADHD can make it challenging to manage your life. Setting goals and achieving them might take a lot of work. Understanding your priorities can help you set goals that align with them and avoid those that are not, making it easier for you to achieve them.

Here are a few steps to get you started:

Step 1:

Which tasks are now your top priorities? Please remember that this may imply saying "not right now" to other things. That's completely alright. You can always return to those later. Make a list of your top three priorities. For example:

1. I'm prioritizing learning new skills.
2. I'm prioritizing my work.
3. I'm prioritizing self-care.

My Top Three Priorities:

1.--

2.--

3.--

Step 2:

To what would you say "not right now," depending on your priorities? What are you doing right now that is diverting attention from your focus? What are you concentrating on? Remember, you're not saying "no," but rather "not right now" to this. You can return to it later when your priorities have changed. For example:

- I spend too long on social media.
- I spend hours binging a TV series.
- I'm trying to learn digital art.

Right now, I'm concentrating on

1.------------------------------

2.------------------------------

3.------------------------------

Step 3:

Now use your priorities to identify goals. For

example,

- I want to learn French.
- I want to be more spiritual.
- I want to get a promotion.

My top three goals are

1.-------------------------------

2.-------------------------------

3.-------------------------------

Step 4:

Develop these goals into SMART goals. For example:

Goal one- I want to learn French.

The elements of SMART goals:

- **Specific**: I wish to speak French fluently to get along with people in France better.

- **Measurable**: I'll take an online lesson once a week and practice with my classmates to measure my improvement.

- **Achievable**: I have prior language learning

experience and some extra time.

- **Relevant**: I wish to speak French because I want to travel to France for vacation.
- **Time-based:** I have a two-month trip to France scheduled.

Complete SMART Goal: I'll begin weekly French lessons next week, practicing with others to improve over the next six months to speak fluently when I visit France.

My first SMART goal

(--)

Goal two- I want to be more spiritual.

The elements of SMART goals:

- **Specific**: I wish to start a daily spiritual practice to improve myself.
- **Measurable**: I'll keep a daily practice journal.
- **Achievable**: I can exercise daily, and I've joined a spiritual community to hold myself accountable.

- **Relevant**: I will now be able to live the better life I have always desired.

- **Time-based**: My journey will begin on April first, and I'll record it for a year before re-evaluating.

Complete SMART Goal: I'll start my daily spiritual practice and join the community on April first. I'll keep a daily journal for a year to record my development and assess my progress.

My second SMART goal

(---)

Step 5:

Although it may be easy to identify your goals, following through with them can be challenging. Now that you've measured and set your goals, compare them to these standard ADHD struggles to check if you could make any changes:

- *Working memory*: Forgetting the primary purpose or its subgoals.

Possible solution: Write down the goals and subgoals to externalize memory issues.

- *Time blindness*: Losing track of time or failing to estimate the duration of a task.

Possible solution: Check the duration of previous tasks of a similar kind, and double it if you're in doubt. Set up visual systems that show you the course of a job.

- *Transition times*: While switching from one task to another, you may need more time to focus on your goals.

Possible solution: Put together similar goal-related tasks. Plan transitions between functions that are not similar.

- *Dopamine*: The feeling that the goals on your list are too dull to begin.

Possible solution: By taking breaks and rewarding yourself at the end of the task, you can make it more tolerable. You can also spice up tedious duties, such as doing chores while listening to music.

Short and Long-term Goals

Prioritizing urgent short-term goals is usually the easiest to achieve with ADHD. Long-term, multi-step goals are tricky. One of the reasons is that things that are "in the future" typically don't feel as urgent and are consequently less motivating. This is why setting subgoals and assigning deadlines for them may be just as important as it is for the primary goal. You can continue to work toward completing your primary goal by achieving these sub-goals.

You set short-term goals for things you wish to accomplish quickly. You could complete it by the end of the day, week, or month, and it could just need a few steps. A short-term goal will allow you to enjoy the rewards quite fast.

Waiting months or years to achieve a long-term goal may seem complicated. Setting several short-term goals along the journey is the key to achieving long-term goals. For example, to become a lawyer, you must finish your undergraduate studies, pass the LSAT and the MPRE, pass the bar, and then be qualified to practice law. However, if you start by setting a goal to apply to law school or college, you may accomplish that sooner.

Tips for Setting Goals

Here are nine tips to help you set your goal with ADHD:

- **Tip one:** Set SMART goals. To set a goal, follow the SMART rule: specific, measurable, achievable, relevant, and time-based.
- **Tip two:** Get organized. It's time to organize and establish a routine once you've determined your goal.
- **Tip three:** Keep it simple. Reduce the number of steps you need to take to accomplish your goal. The more steps there are, the more likely you won't do it.
- **Tip four:** Set alarms and reminders. Put your routine and the planned steps into your calendar and set alarms for them. Set multiple alarms if you tend to ignore them.
- **Tip five:** Make it entertaining. You'll be more likely to complete the task if it's enjoyable.
- **Tip six:** Find a partner for accountability. Find someone who will hold you responsible for conducting your tasks, whether it be a friend, partner, coworker, or even a group.
- **Tip seven:** Treat yourself to healthy rewards. Reward yourself whenever you complete a

task, but do it healthily.

- **Tip eight:** Re-evaluate if you need help achieving your goal. Ask yourself these questions: Do I care about the outcome? Are the tasks taking longer than I expected? Am I trying to accomplish my goal at a moment that doesn't favour me? Is my strategy failing? Do I care too much about doing things correctly even to begin?

- **Tip nine:** Seek help and feedback. Share your goals, strengths, and areas of weakness with others. Then, ask for their input and support.

Live Healthy

One of the best ways to deal with ADHD is to have a healthy mindset and body. Here are quick tips for a healthy lifestyle:

- Regularly consume a balanced diet rich in whole foods such as fruits, vegetables, and whole grains.
- Being active and getting a lot of exercise during the day.
- Sleeping for at least seven hours.
- Taking daily walks or other outdoor activities.
- Maintaining a clutter-free environment.
- Limiting screen time, such as TV, laptops,

tablets, and smartphones.

- Setting alarms and reminders for important dates or tasks.
- Instead of multitasking, work on one thing at a time.
- Limiting distractions like keeping your phone out of reach.
- Making notes of your symptoms and experiences in a journal or notebook.

With time and experience, you can establish techniques to help you strengthen your focus and regulate your impulses.

◆ ◆ ◆

Key Takeaways

- The symptoms of ADHD include inattentiveness, hyperactivity, impulsivity, and difficulties with executive function.
- ADHD can impact all areas of your life, from your relationships and career to your physical and emotional health.
- Various treatments are available for ADHD, including medication, therapy, lifestyle changes, and alternative approaches.
- Understanding and accepting your diagnosis is essential to manage your symptoms and improving your quality of life.
- Setting clear goals, creating structure and routine, and utilizing organizational tools can help you manage the symptoms of ADHD.
- With the right strategies and mindset, it's possible to live a fulfilling and successful life with ADHD.

If you found this chapter helpful, you'll want to read the next chapter, "Understanding ADHD with Women." This chapter focuses on the unique challenges women with ADHD face. It provides practical strategies for managing symptoms and thriving in daily life. From accepting yourself to self-compassion and meditation, you'll find valuable insights to help you navigate life with ADHD as a woman. So don't wait–dive into the next chapter and continue your journey to thriving with adult ADHD.

◆ ◆ ◆

CHAPTER 2: UNDERSTANDIN G ADHD WITH WOMEN

> *ADHD in women is like juggling a million things while walking on a tightrope. It takes a toll on mental and emotional health. –Dr. Kathleen Nadeau*

Women with ADHD are often overlooked and misunderstood. Many women go undiagnosed or misdiagnosed for years, struggling to resolve their challenges. This chapter will cover the unique challenges and experiences of women with ADHD, including cultivating an acceptance mentality and practicing self-compassion.

We will also explore the common symptoms of

ADHD in women and how they can impact your daily life. Finally, we will discuss the benefits of meditation and other mindfulness practices in managing ADHD symptoms and promoting overall well-being.

ADHD is more commonly diagnosed in men than women. Women are less likely to engage in disruptive behaviour, which can accentuate the symptoms of ADHD, and is more likely to exhibit signs of inattentiveness. This implies that women with ADHD are rarely diagnosed. Unfortunately, women are more likely to internalize and blame themselves for their perceived shortcomings. As a result, they suffer from depression.

Women who are impulsive or inattentive often believe that "something" is wrong with them. As they grow up, shame and guilt might ingrain into their personality. After receiving the first diagnosis of ADHD, they might experience a sense of relief and even exhilaration for being able to give it a name. However, a diagnosis cannot change inherent personality traits.

The real work begins after the diagnosis. They must comprehensively understand how ADHD impacts their unique strengths and weaknesses. Women with this disorder may find that the condition has certain benefits. Their enthusiasm and spontaneity may turn the home into a haven for the children. Their high energy may help them simultaneously manage a demanding job and a hectic personal life.

Some women consider treatment for ADHD because their lives are out of control. They may struggle to keep up with the demands of their jobs, their finances may be in crisis mode, and they may feel even less capable of managing day-to-day duties. Other women are more skilled in hiding their ADHD, working tirelessly to meet expectations. However, regardless of how well-hidden their troubles are or how chaotic their life appears, they frequently describe themselves as overwhelmed and drained.

Dysphoria, severe depression, and anxiety disorders are common in women with ADHD. They appear to have lower self-image and higher psychological distress than men with the same diagnosis. Compared to neurotypical women, women diagnosed with ADHD in adulthood are more likely to have depressive symptoms, are more stressed and anxious, have lower self-esteem, and tend to engage in more emotional coping mechanisms than task-oriented ones.

Women with ADHD suffer from the physical and psychological effects of chronic stress. According to studies, having a family member with ADHD causes stress for the entire family. However, women can also experience higher stress levels because they are more responsible for the house and children than men. Inadequate diagnosis and treatment of ADHD in women is a severe public health issue.

Finding a professional to offer effective treatment can be tricky, even for women lucky enough to get a proper diagnosis. Few doctors have expertise in treating adult ADHD, and even fewer are knowledgeable of the particular difficulties faced by women showing symptoms. As a result, the majority of doctors adopt standard psychotherapy techniques. Although these methods can help shed light on emotional and interpersonal problems, they do not assist women with ADHD in learning how to manage their condition better daily or lead more productive and fulfilling lives.

Developing Acceptance Mentality

To reduce the effects of ADHD, it is also essential to establish strategies that can be followed at home without the assistance of a therapist, coach, or organizer.

◆ ◆ ◆

Date ---------

Exercise 4

The following techniques can be applied at home, without the guidance of an expert, which might be helpful for a woman with ADHD, please reflect on each one in the space below:

- Instead of criticizing and blaming yourself, understand and accept the difficulties caused by your ADHD.

- Find the sources of stress in your everyday life, then gradually change your lifestyle to minimize stress.

- Make your life simpler.

- Ask relatives and friends for guidance and support.

- Consult with parenting experts.

- Make your family ADHD-friendly by encouraging cooperation and mutual support.

- Make time for yourself every day.

- Establish healthy habits for your well-being by getting enough sleep, exercising, and eating well.

- Pay attention to what you enjoy.

ADHD and Women

There is currently very little known about ADHD in women because there has been so little research on this particular group of people. Women have recently started receiving ADHD diagnoses and treatment; therefore, most of what we now know about this population is based on the clinical experience of mental health experts specializing in treating women.

Women with ADHD are usually not diagnosed when they are younger and are not identified until they are adults. More often than not, a woman recognizes her own ADHD symptoms after one of her children is diagnosed. She starts recognizing many of the same tendencies as she learns more about her child's condition.

Even though research on adult females with ADHD lags behind men's, many physicians are discovering problematic issues and co-existing disorders in females with ADHD. Women with ADHD may also struggle with compulsive eating, alcoholism, and chronic sleep deprivation. Major depression, anxiety disorders, and dysphoria are also common in women with ADHD, similar to men. However, compared to men with ADHD, women seem to have lower self-esteem and experience more severe psychological distress.

ADHD impacts multiple aspects of emotion, cognition, behaviours and day-to-day functioning. A multimodal strategy that involves medication, psychotherapy, stress management, and ADHD coaching could be used to treat adult women struggling with their symptoms. Self-esteem, interpersonal and familial concerns, daily lifestyle habits, level of stress, and life management skills are some topics addressed by ADHD-focused therapy. These treatments are frequently called "neurocognitive psychotherapy," a combination of cognitive behaviour therapy and rehabilitation methods. Cognitive rehabilitation focuses on life management skills (remembering, reasoning, understanding, problem-solving, and evaluating).

In contrast, cognitive behaviour therapy focuses on the psychological concerns of ADHD (self-esteem, self-acceptance, and self-blame).

Even with proper diagnosis and treatment, women with ADHD often get negative feedback as they balance relationships with their families, friends, and others. They are often told by themselves or others that they are too much, frustrating, lazy, uninspired, not living up to their full potential, demanding, irritating, or weird.

A woman with ADHD builds her identity and sense of self on these labels and interactions with others. Everyone must learn to love, understand, and accept themselves. Still, women with this disorder may need extra support and encouragement to do so in a more organized and structured way.

Daily Issues (ADHD Symptoms)

Try to look past the problematic ADHD symptoms and discover the "mirror qualities" or the positive aspects of the ADHD symptoms. For example, although many women with ADHD appear hyperactive, they might also be considered energetic. Instead of being labelled stubborn, a woman with ADHD might be considered persistent. A young girl may battle impulsivity while being perceived as creative and spontaneous. What we see in the mirror varies depending on where we are standing.

◆ ◆ ◆

Date ---------

Exercise 5

Considering the challenges they create in the following five main aspects, you may better understand how deeply executive function issues, poor self-control, and poor inhibition affect your life. To understand how ADHD affects you, quickly check the challenges you have experienced:

Poor goal-setting, time management, and planning

- Do you procrastinate or wait until the last minute to complete tasks?

- Do you frequently miss assignment due dates?

- Do you need help making plans or getting prepared for upcoming events?

- Do you find it challenging to manage multiple tasks at once?

- Do you need help estimating the duration of a job or how long it will take to go somewhere?

- Do you struggle to manage your finances?

- Do you need help finding the motivation to begin or finish a task?

Suppose you have experienced a considerable number of these issues. In that case, it should be clear that ADHD in adults is a difficulty with the ability to organize activity over time to prepare for the future.

Poor self-organization, problem-solving, and working memory

- Do you find it difficult to do mental calculations?

- Do you need help to think clearly or organize your thoughts?

- When talking to people, do you often need to remember the point you were trying to make?

- Do you think people with similar intelligence are more imaginative or creative than you?

- Do you need help to pick up new or challenging tasks as quickly as others?

- Do you work to carry out tasks in the correct order or sequence?

- Do you take longer to respond to unexpected events?

From personal experience, you may already know that people with ADHD have significant difficulties organizing their thoughts and activities quickly and efficiently and coming up with different solutions to daily challenges.

Poor self-discipline (Inhibition)

- Do you frequently make impulsive decisions?

- Do you find it difficult to stop your activities or behaviour when you should?

- Do you often say things out of the blue to

other people?

- Do you tend to act without thinking about the consequences?

- Do you make last-minute plans on a whim or an impulse?

- Do you consider the future less than other people your age appear to?

- Do you find it difficult to be objective about issues affecting you?

- Are you highly picky about how things should be done?

- Are you easily irritated or angered?

Not only do these inhibition issues affect behaviour, but also thought and emotion. This is why lack of inhibition has such a wide-ranging impact on your life. If you can control your impulses long enough for self-discipline and time to take hold, it will drive you to choose the best choices for your long-term well-being.

Poor self-motivation

- If your job is tedious or complex, are you more likely to leave early?

- Do you need to delay gratification or put off activities that are rewarding right now to achieve a future goal?

- Do you need to pay more attention to details when working?

- Do others ever describe you as being unmotivated or lazy?

- Do you need an immediate reward to complete tasks?

- Do you struggle to resist the impulse to do something fun or more engaging when you should be working?

- Do you find it challenging to work as effectively as others without constant supervision or instruction?

You understand how difficult it can be to continue when what you have to do is tedious, requires much work, or is time-consuming. With ADHD, you become dependent on instant gratification or externally imposed consequences. You have to motivate yourself to keep on going.

Poor self-activation, focus, and alertness

- When focusing on anything, are you easily distracted by other thoughts?

- Do you often need to carefully read or listen to the instructions before you start a task or project?

- Do you find it hard to stay awake and attentive in boring situations?

- Are you quickly excited by things happening around you?

- Do you need help maintaining attention when reading, writing, listening or working?

When there is no instant reward, adults with ADHD find it extremely difficult to stay alert, fully engaged, and active to maintain focus.

◆ ◆ ◆

Self-Compassion for ADHD Minds

The idea of self-compassion is straightforward. Mentally, we do not treat ourselves as well as we would like a close friend or young child.

That situation has real-world repercussions and can damage our sense of self, level of confidence, and overall happiness. Self-compassion is a practical remedy for perfectionism and self-criticism.

Having a sense of self-compassion enhances our feelings, problem-solving abilities, resilience, and interpersonal relationships. We learn to prioritize self-improvement and take accountability for our mistakes without internal shaming.

You may have an important meeting, lock yourself out of your apartment, and the key is inside. What comes to your mind first? You will likely think, "What a fool I am; I always mess up, and nothing ever works out."

Now consider seeing your best friend go through the same thing: an important meeting, locked door, key inside. What feelings do you have about your friend's mistake? "Everyone does that, so it is fine! Take your time; everything will be fine." With practice, we can offer the same compassion to ourselves as we would to troubled friends.

It is a myth that having a perfectionist and judgmental mindset keeps us motivated. It is challenging to reach perfection; by pursuing it, we lose our motivation, preventing us from recovering. Success requires the desire to progress and the room to fail, reorganize, and move ahead. A strong attitude is based on the belief that our efforts count. What advice would you give a kid? You made a mistake. What can we do moving forward? This systematic approach makes more room for development, problem-solving, and serious effort. With practice, we can create a more balanced view of ourselves, our lives, and our ADHD.

Self-compassion and mindfulness help women with ADHD by allowing them to understand that negative self-concept and self-doubt are habits rather than hard-wired psychological traits. The three components of an essential self-compassion practice are mindfulness, connection with others, and actively developing a more positive self-perspective.

Not everything needs to be perfect to be "mindful." Being mindful involves paying attention to the present moment and accepting life. It also entails acknowledging our feelings of sadness, and that is all right. Otherwise, we shut down or act out in ways motivated by denial, fear, or wrath.

Connection with others helps in the development of resilience. Whether we have ADHD or not, our problems often cause us to feel odd and isolated in our shortcomings. We are the only ones who make mistakes. We all struggle with something, whether we have ADHD or not. Reminding ourselves that everyone works is the second step in the self-compassion practice. We gain from a sense of belonging.

The final element of the practice is to begin treating yourself like a close friend. We must keep our intentions positive for ourselves and consider how we treat a friend in a similar circumstance. Not that we are perfect or do not need to make improvements, but we can fight the little voice of self-criticism.

Date ---------

Exercise 6

Like with other forms of mindfulness, the overarching goal is to build qualities via repetition. You practice helping ingrain a new way of thinking. There are two ways to approach this exercise. One strategy is to **set a timer** for a few minutes (anything between 5-15 minutes would work), then follow the guidelines for breathing techniques:

- **Step 1:** Find a comfortable position to sit or lie down. If you are seated, try to be focused and upright. Close your eyes or direct your attention to something uninteresting.

- **Step 2:** Take a few deep breaths. Draw your attention, which could be distracted by any other emotion. For now, concentrate on how your body moves with each deep breath.

- **Step 3:** Next, pay attention to each inhale. Take into account the fact that everyone has these moments. You may tell yourself, "This is how I feel right now."

- **Step 4:** Set an intention with each exhalation: "May I find courage and compassion for myself right now." Use any expression that seems natural and that you would use to soothe a friend.
- **Step 5:** Our minds operate in such a way that we will start getting distracted almost immediately. Treat those distractions similarly–accept them as natural, do not get upset, and return to taking your next breath.
- **Step 6:** Continue for a few more breaths or until your timer turns off.

You can use this breathing technique anywhere to relax your body and relieve the anxiety that occasionally comes with ADHD. Over time, it gets easier, especially when coupled with daily meditation. However, you can adjust your perspective at any time. Remind yourself for a few breaths: "Right now, amid this tension, may I stay strong, focused, and gentle to myself."

◆ ◆ ◆

Meditation and ADHD

It may seem contradictory to meditate mindfully when you have the distinct inattentiveness of ADHD. However, according to researchers, it all depends on your strategy. You tell yourself to sit, work, and finish but end up scrolling, standing, and roaming. Behavioural therapies are a viable alternative to medication for the treatment of ADHD.

Mindful meditation offers a simple and easy technique to improve the capacity to complete tasks, pay attention, and reduce stress. A 2017 study indicated that people with ADHD who used mindfulness exercises, such as meditation, performed better in controlling their emotions than those on the trial's waitlist (Mitchell et al., 2013). By training you to accept the discomfort, meditation can help with dopamine deficiency. The best meditation technique for ADHD includes the following steps:

Step 1: Ground yourself

Try grounding yourself at the start of any meditation to prevent mental floatiness. Think about improving your relationship with your physical surroundings by:

- Paying attention to the ground or whatever

you are sitting on.

- Going barefoot to experience the sensation of feeling grounded fully.
- Take a little extra time to thoroughly wash your hands in warm water to appreciate the sensation.

Step 2: Observe your thoughts
When you meditate, your thoughts are scattered. It may be helpful to remember the following:

- It is inevitable for the mind to wander.
- It only gets worse if you criticize your lack of attentiveness.
- You progress in meditation when you become aware of your wandering thoughts.

Step 3: Body scan

Scanning the body might help the mind focus on what it wishes to avoid. Check your shoulders or jaw to see whether they are tense. How does it feel and look? If you notice a place that hurts, you could take a deep breath to ease the pain; however, if you cannot, do not worry.

Step 4: Addressing derailment

- Compassion is the best approach to dealing with your racing thoughts while meditating.
- Pay attention to how your abdomen

expands during inhalation and contracts during exhalation.
- She was chanting or reciting a mantra.
- You are focusing on a tea light to create a focal point. Bring your wandering ideas back to your breath, body, or surrounding space.

You do not have to dramatically change yourself to engage in "behavioural modification" for your ADHD. Mindful meditation is a gentler way to learn to accept your symptoms to increase flow and attention.

ADHD and Hormonal Changes in Women

Researchers are only now beginning to understand whether there is a connection between ADHD and hormones, specifically sex hormones such as Estrogen. Specialists have suggested that there may be a link. After all, many studies have been done on how estrogen levels throughout a woman's life impact her mood and behaviour. However, growing evidence suggests that sex hormones may impact dysfunctional brain circuits in people with ADHD (Mowlem et al., 2018).

ADHD and Estrogen

The reproductive system relies mainly on Estrogen, the predominant sex hormone in women. However, there is a link between Estrogen and other cognitive functions. Several neurotransmitters contribute to ADHD because of their significant impacts on mood, memory, and attention. Dopamine, serotonin, and norepinephrine are all influenced by Estrogen.

Studies have shown that attention and executive functioning skills improve when Estrogen increases (Mowlem et al., 2018). However, when estrogen levels are reduced, symptoms of ADHD might get worse. Estrogen levels fluctuate throughout a woman's life. Besides that, estrogen levels rise and fall every month during the reproductive years. In other words, how symptoms are experienced and treated might depend on how these hormonal changes affect women with ADHD.

Puberty

The hormonal changes throughout puberty result in significant change and emotional instability. Between the ages of 9 and 13, girls often experience physical and emotional changes associated with puberty. There is also a substantial rise in Estrogen and progesterone hormones. It is understandable to assume that girls with ADHD will have an easier time during puberty if their estrogen levels are higher. However, it is usually the other way around. This is because, although Estrogen helps improve ADHD symptoms, progesterone does not. Therefore, keeping a journal for symptoms and talking with your doctor about any changes or problems may be helpful.

Menstruation

Women menstruate every month from puberty till perimenopause, and Estrogen and progesterone levels change over this 28-day menstrual cycle. Although these changes are not as severe as during puberty, they impact ADHD symptoms. It has also been suggested that women with ADHD are more likely to suffer from premenstrual syndrome (PMS).

Pregnancy

Similar to periods and puberty, pregnancy causes a significant change in hormone levels. Throughout the first trimester, ADHD symptoms worsen for many women. The increased progesterone might be responsible, although medication may also be a factor. The first trimester can change significantly since many pregnant women have stopped using their prescribed medication.

There is very little evidence on medication usage and pregnancy-related ADHD. However, there was a difference in mood and social functioning between women who stopped taking medication and those who maintained it. Further study is required to investigate the links.

Menopause

Women start to go through perimenopause at the age of 40. Estrogen levels begin to fall at this point, and menstruation becomes more irregular. This phase can extend up to ten years until menopause. Menopause often causes memory loss, difficulty concentrating, and hot flashes. This can be especially tough for women with ADHD who struggle with focus and attention.

◆ ◆ ◆

Date ---------

Exercise 7

Managing Hormones

Start **tracking the emotions** you experience at each stage of your menstrual cycle. You can use this to confirm whether your mood swings are related to your period. Understanding why you feel so down might help put things into perspective and provide comfort.

Keeping a detailed record of your previous cycles is also helpful if you want to discuss your symptoms with your doctor. Also, it might help your doctor understand the situation better. You can use a period tracking app to monitor your symptoms and cycle.

You can also download or design your chart. Write the day of the month on the top (1 through 31). On the left side of the page, list your symptoms. Mark the checkbox next to the symptoms you experience daily with an 'X.' Note how severe, moderate, or mild each symptom is.

To keep track of your mood swings, make a note of the following symptoms:

- Sadness
- Sudden shifts in mood
- Crying spells
- Trouble focusing
- Little or excessive sleep
- Loss of interest in regular tasks
- Lethargy

◆ ◆ ◆

EXERCISE#7

MANAGING HORMONES

Date:-------

	Symptoms		
	Sadness	Crying spells	Trouble focusing
Day 1	◯ Severe ◯ Moderate ◯ Mild		
Day 2			
Day 3			
Day 4			
Day 5			
Day 6			
Day 7			

Hormonal birth control

Bloating, tender breasts, and other physical PMS symptoms can be treated using hormonal birth control methods like pills or patches. They may also help some people with emotional symptoms like mood swings. However, for some people, hormonal birth control might trigger mood swings. If you choose this course, you might have to experiment with different birth control options until you find one suitable.

Natural remedies

Vitamins help with PMS-related mood swings. A calcium supplement was proven to help with PMS-related depression, frustration, and anxiety. Calcium-rich foods include milk, yogurt, cheese, leafy green vegetables, fortified orange juice, and cereal. Vitamin B-6 may also help with PMS symptoms, and it is found in fruit, fortified cereals, fish, chicken, and turkey.

Lifestyle changes

- **Exercise**: Try to be active for at least 30 minutes weekly. Regular walking in your area might ease sadness, anger, or stress.

- **Nutrition**: When PMS hits, try to avoid junk food. Excessive amounts of sugar, fat, and salt might all harm your mood. Try to balance these meals with fruits, vegetables, and whole grains. This will help you stay full throughout the day and minimize blood sugar fluctuations, which can make you irritable.

- **Sleep**: Sleep for at least seven to eight hours every night, especially the week before your period. If your period is only days away, lack of sleep might make you miserable. Figure out what happens to your body and mind when you do not get enough sleep.

- **Stress**: Having stress might make mood swings worse. Try deep breathing techniques, meditation, or yoga to relax your mind and body, especially when encountering PMS symptoms.

◆ ◆ ◆

Key Takeaways

- ADHD affects women differently than men and is often under or misdiagnosed in women.
- Women with ADHD may struggle with emotional regulation, time management, organization, and relationships.
- Hormonal fluctuations can exacerbate ADHD symptoms during the menstrual cycle, pregnancy, and menopause.
- Practicing self-compassion and self-care can help women with ADHD manage their symptoms and improve their quality of life.
- Developing effective coping strategies, such as mindfulness and meditation, can help women with ADHD reduce stress and improve emotional regulation.
- Women with ADHD can thrive personally and professionally with the proper support and tools, such as medication, therapy, and organizational techniques.

If you are ready to take your understanding of ADHD to the next level, do not miss the next chapter on "Understanding Executive Function with ADHD," where you will gain valuable insights into how your brain works and how you can improve your executive function skills. Get ready to unlock your potential and thrive with ADHD.

◆ ◆ ◆

CHAPTER 3: UNDERSTAND EXECUTIVE FUNCTION WITH ADHD

ADHD is a neurological condition that affects executive functions, such as planning, organizing, and decision-making. –Dr. Roberto Olivardia

Executive function is like the CEO of your brain, responsible for managing and coordinating all the different mental processes that help you achieve your goals. However, for women with ADHD, executive function can feel like a constant battle. This chapter will explore what executive function is and how ADHD can impact it.

We will dive into the different domains of executive function, from planning and organization to emotional regulation and impulse control. By the end of this chapter, you will better understand how executive function affects your daily life and how to strengthen your skills in this crucial area.

As discussed earlier, women with executive dysfunctions, such as ADHD, often experience time blindness or the inability to organize and remember upcoming events. They also need help to coordinate their actions to achieve long-term goals. This is an executive functioning issue rather than a difficulty with attention. A woman struggling with executive functioning may struggle to analyze, plan, organize, schedule, and complete tasks.

Women with executive dysfunction usually struggle with managing their emotions, starting and completing tasks, memorizing and following instructions that include several stages, staying on topic, self-monitoring, and balancing tasks. The principal executive functions are:

- **Working memory:** Working memory is the memory that is associated with what you are doing right now. Your working memory is used when you are reading, taking notes, or having a conversation.

- **Cognitive flexibility:** This is sometimes called fluid, or flexible, thinking and describes how easily your mind can switch between different topics. The more flexible your thinking, the better you adjust to your surroundings. This helps you in reacting to sudden changes. People with more flexible thought processes are often incredibly imaginative and creative. This skill enables people to link concepts and ideas that otherwise seem unrelated.
- **Inhibition control:** The ability to guide or direct your thoughts, emotions, and behaviours is called inhibition control. Without it, we could not regulate our impulses and thoughts. Inhibition control functions in two ways:

    - *Behaviour control* is the ability to restrain yourself from acting in ways you believe you should not. Keeping quiet around someone who is highly unpleasant is one example of this.

    - *Attention control* is the ability to direct or control your thought processes. It involves focusing on what requires your attention and ignoring what does not. Sometimes your concentration and focus are outside your mind. You may need to use distraction control to prevent your thoughts from diverting your attention.

Executive function is built on working memory, cognitive flexibility, and inhibitory control. However, other higher-level processes can occur, such as:

- **Planning:** This is when you create a mental plan for a series of steps to enable you to complete a task.

- **Reasoning:** This is the ability for critical thinking. You must build on your acquired knowledge and think imaginatively or split something difficult into manageable parts.

- **Problem-solving:** This function may include all three primary executive functions, planning and reasoning. This is how you use what you know and how you think to overcome obstacles or challenges.

Part of the Brain That Controls Executive Functions

The brain's executive function controls and facilitates the application of behaviour and skills. This enables us to do time management, self-control, planning, flexible thinking, and organizing.

In general, executive functioning is stimulated whenever we are required to take action, correct mistakes, make plans, or strive to overcome impulses. The frontal lobe mainly regulates these executive functions, that is, the prefrontal regions, such as the prefrontal cortex.

These are linked to the cortical, subcortical, and brainstem regions. It will not affect your verbal or cognitive functions even if you have prefrontal damage. Instead, it impacts the connections linking it to other brain parts.

The prefrontal cortex covers the first part of the frontal lobe. This part of the brain is responsible for planning actions, regulating social behaviour, expressing personality, and making decisions. We use it to direct our activities and thoughts toward our goals. This part allows learning specific rules compared to other parts of the brain. With abstraction, anterior regions help rule learning.

The prefrontal cortex's function is to help you focus, think about the consequences of your choices, control impulsive behaviour and emotional reactions, plan for the future, and regulate complex behaviours. A delayed emotional response can occur when the prefrontal cortex is injured. As a result, a person is more likely to make poor judgments.

It is essential to understand the significance of the frontal lobe in executive functioning and how significant these functions are in our lives. The prefrontal cortex is divided into three regions. The medial part is involved with motivation and attention.

The orbital part allows you to control distractions while controlling urges. The lateral part enables the development and execution of plans. Once we fully understand the importance of the prefrontal cortex, we will understand how essential it is to take good care of it and ensure it functions correctly.

Examples of Executive Dysfunction

Because executive functions involve so many activities within the brain, they can manifest in several ways:

- They are easily distracted or need help with concentrating on a single activity.
- Excessive focus on a single topic.
- Zoning out while you should be paying attention.
- Having trouble visualizing the outcome or goal of an action makes it difficult to plan or complete it.

- I need help getting myself to start an activity that seems complicated or tedious.
- I need help to switch from one activity to another.
- Losing focus as a result of being interrupted or distracted mid-task.
- Problems controlling impulses.
- You struggle to think things through before you speak, so you tend to say whatever comes to mind without considering whether it would offend someone.
- You understand your thought process in your brain, but it feels difficult to put it into words for other people. This makes it challenging to communicate your thought process properly.

Executive Function Skills

We use our executive function skills daily to manage our lives and achieve our goals. They help us achieve important goals like building a career, buying a house, or earning a degree. They also help us achieve small goals, such as getting ready for a job interview, finishing a project at work, and handling daily responsibilities.

◆◆◆

Date ---------

Exercise 8

This exercise will help you understand your executive skills, strengths, and weaknesses. If you can find ways to build on your strengths and improve the challenging areas, you can do better at achieving your goals.

After reading each item:

1. Score it based on how much you agree or disagree with how well it defines you.
2. Choose the ideal score using the rating scale.
3. After you have completed all 24 questions, please write down your scores for each of them and add the scores from each section.

There are three questions in each section. Note down the skills with the highest and lowest score.

We all face different challenges. Knowing our strengths and weaknesses helps us consider how we can use our strengths to overcome our shortcomings or improve the skills we are struggling with so they will not prevent us from reaching our goals.

Although it is not a formal test, you can show it to your healthcare professional to outline your skill base and condition so they can develop a more effective treatment strategy to improve your skill set.
Rating scale:

- 1 = Strongly disagree
- 2 = Disagree
- 3 = Tend to disagree
- 4 = Tend to agree
- 5 = Agree
- 6 = Strongly agree

Working Memory

1. I can recall details, dates, and information with ease.

My score is ( )

2. I am good at keeping track of what I need to accomplish.

My score is ( )

3. I rarely need reminders to complete tasks.

My score is ( )

My total score for this section ( )

Emotional Control

1. I never let my emotions keep me from accomplishing tasks.

My score is ( )

2. I do not let little things bother me or stop me from doing what needs to be done.

My score is ( )

3. I do not lose my temper when I am upset or irritated.

My score is ( )

My total score for this section ( )

Planning

1. I have a clear plan for what to do when I start my day.

My score is ( )

2. I can easily focus on essential tasks despite too many pending tasks.

My score is ( )

3. I often divide big tasks into smaller ones and set deadlines.

My score is ( )

My total score for this section ( )

Organization

1. I like to keep everything in order.

My score is ( )

2. I usually keep my workspace tidy and

organized.

My score is ( )

3. I am skilled at organizing my work.

My score is ( )

My total score for this section ( )

Flexibility

1. Unexpected events do not bother me.

My score is ( )

2. I am easily adaptable to changes in plans.

My score is ( )

3. I am flexible and versatile.

My score is ( )

My total score for this section ( )

Reasoning

1. I regularly assess my performance and find ways to get better.

My score is ( )

2. I can step back from a situation and make an objective decision.

My score is ( )

3. I like to think about the "big picture" and enjoy the problem-solving that comes with it.

My score is ( )

My total score for this section ( )

Behaviour control

1. I refrain from making quick judgments.

My score is ( )

2. I think before I speak.

My score is ( )

3. Before I act, I make sure I am fully informed.

My score is ( )

My total score for this section ( )

Sustained attention

1. I have no trouble maintaining focus while working.

My score is ( )

2. I work persistently until a project or assignment is finished.

My score is ( )

3. I find it easy to resume and complete my work after being interrupted and complete it.

My score is ( )

My total score for this section ( )

Activities to Improve Executive Function Skills

Practice is essential for improving any executive function. It flourishes most effectively when we reduce the factors that hinder executive functioning (such as stress) and increase the factors that nurture it (like happiness or feelings of belonging). In order to improve, executive functions need to be consistently evaluated. However, the best outcomes will only be achieved through training and practice.

◆ ◆ ◆

Date --------

Exercise 9

There are three primary executive functioning skills:

Working memory

It is the capacity to store knowledge in the mind and use it later. Working memory differs from short-term memory, which stores information without using it. Working memory allows us to:

- Mentally play with thoughts and connect one idea to the next.
- Think about the past or the future.
- Remember to follow multi-step instructions in the correct order.
- Remember a question while focusing on the ongoing conversation.
- Make logical sense of everything that changes over time, which involves remembering the past and connecting it to the present.

Things you can do to improve working memory:

- Mentally calculate things like discounts or

total costs while shopping or scores during a game.

- Play a memory game that requires one person to tell a story, the next person to repeat it and add to it, and so on.
- Listening to stories because it challenges the listener's working memory to recall all of the story's details and link them to new information as the story develops.
- Reciting speeches or slam poetry helps improve working memory and attention skills.

Cognitive flexibility

Cognitive flexibility comprises the following abilities:

- Consider a problem or situation from different angles. It is considering things from several perspectives. For example, consider an alternative viewpoint or a different approach to an issue.
- Take a fresh look at something.
- Take advantage of a rare opportunity.
- Find a solution to overcome challenges or unforeseen issues.
- After learning new facts, acknowledge you were mistaken before.
- Adapt to change or the unexpected.

Things you can do to improve cognitive flexibility:

- Participate in improvisational activities, such as dancing and painting, which helps nurture and stimulate creativity and make quick adjustments.
- Play games that require creative thinking.
- Find unique uses for everyday items.
- For example, vinegar may be used for cooking, cleaning, or weed control.
- Play a game involving finding similarities between ordinary things. For example: How are tomatoes similar to oranges? (In terms of shape or colour.)

Inhibition control

Behaviour control

The ability to resist temptation, think things through before speaking or acting, and control impulses are examples of inhibitory behaviour control. Inhibitory control is necessary for discipline and persistence, which include putting off pleasure or staying on task despite difficulties. Activities to improve inhibitory control of behaviour:

- Performing for a dramatic play to practice inhibiting acting out of character.
- Playing music with others develops the

ability to wait for your turn to play.

- Putting up a comedy act to practice not laughing at your jokes.

Attention control

The capacity to put aside distractions to concentrate, pay attention, and maintain that focus even when the subject is boring. Some activities to improve inhibitory control of attention:

- Singing in a group is the ultimate exercise for assessing inhibitory control of attention.
- Reading aloud should enhance sustained attention because it forces listeners to work harder to focus without visual aids.
- Walking in a straight line requires both balance and focused attention.
- I was walking with a bell and trying not to make it ring. It is also effective for de-stressing.
- Activities include pouring a drink, carrying a tray full of filled glasses, juggling and stitching, challenging fine and gross motor skills, and focusing attention and concentration.

Self-Reflection and ADHD

Attention Deficit/Hyperactivity Disordered brains lean far too much toward magical thinking. We want things to change, but we want them to change without any continued effort on our part.

Alternatively, we resist our ADHD brains, denying and rejecting truths about how we function correctly. The core problem with this disorder is the transition from knowing to doing. Knowing what to do is different from actually doing it.

Real change and progress can only happen when we accept ourselves and recognize the differences in our ADHD. The more self-aware we become and understand who we are, the easier it is to utilize our strengths and find solutions when necessary. Understanding and using our cognitive abilities are essential for planning and acting productively. The more we understand the process, the easier it becomes.

The first step in developing self-awareness is to list your strengths and weaknesses, including who you are, what you are likely to do, and how you work versus how you wish you worked. Without self-awareness, you risk creating a life or engaging in actions that will not benefit you. Knowing who you are and how you function can help you develop strategies to enhance your skills and compensate for your ADHD difficulties. For example, when you know what makes you angry, you can take action to ease those feelings.

◆ ◆ ◆

Date ---------

Exercise 10

Some countless questions and exercises can be used for self-reflection. Some questions can be asked, addressed, and resolved daily, while others would be reserved for occasional self-reflection. To get some ideas for reflective questions, go through the following lists:

To get your self-reflection started, try these ten questions:

1. Am I making the most of my time?
   ✓ ....
   ✗ ....
2. Is there anything I take for granted?
   ✓ ....
   ✗ ....
3. Am I adopting a positive outlook?
   ✓ ....
   ✗ ....
4. Am I being genuine in my life?
   ✓ ....
   ✗ ....
5. Do I get up in the morning feeling ready to face the day?

✓ ....

✕ ....

6. Do I get negative thoughts before I go to sleep?

✓ ....

✕ ....

7. Do I invest enough time and energy in my relationships?

✓ ....

✕ ....

8. Am I looking after my physical needs?

✓ ....

✕ ....

9. Do I become stressed out by things that are beyond my control?

✓ ....

✕ ....

10. Are the goals I have set for myself being met?

✓ ....

✕ ....

You can ask yourself the following ten questions every day to learn more about yourself:

1. What about the future worries me the most?

....

....

2. What am I afraid of?

....

....

3. Am I clinging to anything that I should let go of?

4. What am I doing about the things that are most important to me?

5. When was the last time I stepped outside of my comfort zone?

6. What should I change about myself?

7. Who has influenced my life the most?

8. Which is worse, not trying at all or failing?

9. Does what other people think of me matter?

10. To what extent have I honestly had control over my life?

Write down your answers after asking yourself these questions. The questions and answers can be as creative as you wish. Ask yourself questions about your past, present, and future, then write inspiring, informative, and motivating answers. There are no "correct" answers, and your answers will probably change over time. Ensure your questions are written in a way that includes specifics about your goals. The more specific your questions and answers are the more potential for in-depth self-reflection.

Journaling

Journaling can be an effective tool for women with ADHD in several ways. It can help them to understand better and manage their symptoms. By reflecting on their thoughts and emotions, women with ADHD can gain insight into what triggers their distractibility, impulsivity, and hyperactivity and develop strategies to cope with them. Journaling can also provide a sense of structure and organization, which can be helpful for people who may struggle with time management and planning.

Journaling has countless benefits and multiple ways to use it for reflection. Journaling can be calming and soothing, helping to reduce anxiety and stress. By creating a safe space to express themselves, women with ADHD may also experience greater self-awareness and self-acceptance. Three things to note in your journal every day:

1. At least one good thing happened to you or someone around you today.
2. Ask yourself one question, but wait to provide an answer. You can use a question from the last exercise, one from the previous lists, or something new.
3. A reflection on the question you asked yourself the day before and a possible answer.

If you follow these instructions, you will only note the first two parts on the first day, but from the next day onward, you will note all three parts every day.

◆ ◆ ◆

Date ---------

Exercise 11

The **worksheets** listed below can be used with questions, prompts, writing suggestions, and exercises to help you start your reflection. This worksheet is a good source of activities and tips to get you to evaluate your skills, traits, values, and beliefs.

This worksheet is divided into multiple sections, each of which includes a unique set of questions and guidelines:

Talent

- What are your best talents or skills?

- Which skills or talents make you feel the proudest or most satisfied?

Traits/ Qualities

- What are your top five qualities?

- What do you consider to be your two most significant flaws?

- What traits do you most appreciate in other people?

Principles

- What ten things stand out to you as truly important?

- What are the top three priorities in your life?

- What are the principles that are most valuable to you?

Perception

- How are the "public you" and the "private you" different?

- What do you want others to say and think about you?

- Is being liked by others more important than being liked by yourself?

Achievement

- What are your three most remarkable accomplishments in your life?

- What goals do you wish to achieve in life?

- What would you do if you could only do one thing before you died?

Reflection

- What (music, animal, flower, sign, etc.) best describes who you are? Why?

- Which three things about yourself would you most like to change?

- Name three characteristics you have.

In the last part, you will be given a variety of possibilities to respond to. Complete the sentence:

- I am at my best when...

- I struggle when...

- I stress when...

- I am brave when...

- One of the most important lessons I learned was...

- I missed an excellent chance when...

- One of my most treasured memories is...

- My most challenging decisions are...

- Being myself is not easy because...

- I want to be more...

- I wish I could...

- I wish I would go regularly...

- I wished I had...

- I wish I felt...

- I wish I knew...

- I wish I had seen it...

- I am going to focus on...

After completing this worksheet, you will understand your true personality and priorities well. Use the information you acquire to help you decide what goals you want to pursue, what you want to accomplish in the future, and what steps to take next.

◆ ◆ ◆

Key Takeaways

- Women with ADHD often experience executive function challenges, impacting their ability to manage time, prioritize tasks, and stay organized.
- Building structure and routine into your daily life can help manage executive function difficulties.
- Breaking down complex tasks into smaller, more manageable ones can make staying focused and motivated easier.
- Using visual aids, such as calendars, to-do lists, and reminder systems can help women with ADHD stay organized and on track.
- Self-awareness and self-compassion can help women with ADHD manage their emotions and reduce stress.

Suppose you found the chapter insightful and empowering. The next chapter, "How to Control My Emotions and Deal With Rejection Efficiently," can help you build on that foundation.

Here, you will learn practical strategies for managing emotions and coping with rejection healthily and effectively. You will discover how to recognize and regulate your emotions, improve your self-esteem, and develop resilience in the face of rejection.

So if you are ready to take the next step in your journey to thriving with ADHD, I highly recommend diving into the next chapter. Let us continue on this path of growth and self-discovery together!

◆ ◆ ◆

CHAPTER 4: HOW TO CONTROL MY EMOTIONS AND DEAL WITH REJECTION EFFICIENTLY?

ADHD can make it challenging to manage the intense emotions of rejection, leading to avoidance and isolation. –Dr. Kathleen Nadeau

Dealing with rejection is tough for anyone, but for women with ADHD, it can feel like an emotional rollercoaster. ADHD can make it hard to regulate your emotions and stay grounded regarding rejection, leading to feelings of overwhelm, anger, or shame.

In this chapter, we will cover a range of strategies to help you better manage your emotions and deal with rejection effectively. We will explore the concept of emotional regulation and how self-reflection can help you better understand and manage your feelings.

You will also learn practical tips for handling rejection efficiently, improving your self-esteem, and managing the hormonal fluctuations that can come with ADHD. By the end of this chapter, you will have a toolkit of skills to help you stay balanced and resilient in the face of emotional challenges.

In the teenage years, hormonal changes significantly affect the neurochemical issues brought on by ADHD. A combination of these dysregulated systems causes severe mood swings, hyper-irritability, and emotional outbursts. Compared to boys, girls with ADHD tend to have more peer-related issues. Impulsive and energetic teenage boys may be seen as just playing around.

They may even get a lot of peer approval when they rebel against authorities or their hard-drinking, fast-driving, sexually active lifestyle. Parents, teachers, and classmates are far more critical of girls than boys. Later in life, as young women, they often echo the remarks of condemnation and anger, blaming themselves and experiencing intense shame for their past actions.

With the best of intentions, parents too often condemn and criticize girls with ADHD. These girls often have low self-esteem, regardless of whether they are outspoken and rebellious or reserved and quiet. Usually, girls with ADHD believe they are suitable for nothing. They get low grades due to their disorganization, impulsivity, and distraction. A home is a crucial place to recharge and repair the self-confidence that is usually damaged throughout the school day.

Similarly, they must acquire skills and talents like their other friends. Helping them discover their talent or aptitude by praising and acknowledging them for it is significant positive reinforcement. When a teenage girl with ADHD finds an activity that makes her feel good about herself, her life usually takes a turn for the better.

Emotional Regulation

Emotions are healthy and natural. Emotional regulation refers to how you feel and communicate your emotions. You can achieve your goals when you control your emotions regardless of how you feel. Emotional regulation is comprised of five processes:

- Choosing circumstances that limit your negative feelings and enhance positive ones.
- In a given situation, control what you can.
- Focusing on the specific parts of an event gives you a positive sense.
- Rethinking unpleasant circumstances.
- Avoid acts that are just motivated by negative feelings and might worsen your situation.

If you have ADHD, the procedures necessary for emotional regulation might not come naturally to you, which could result in emotional dysregulation. This includes not being able to control your emotions to achieve your goals. Emotions can be heightened by impulsivity and executive function difficulties. Anger, frustration, and impatience can strike suddenly, intensely, and for a prolonged period.

Emotional dysregulation, especially in emotional responses, is common in women with ADHD. As people age, the correlation between emotional dysregulation and the disorder increases. Adults with ADHD may experience issues due to emotional dysregulation, such as interpersonal issues, frustration with other drivers, and car accidents.

Instead of being the cause of the primary symptoms of ADHD, it appears to be their source.

However, suppose you have ADHD and difficulty regulating your emotions. In that case, you are more likely to face challenges than if you only have ADHD with attention and hyperactivity symptoms.

◆ ◆ ◆

Date ---------

Exercise 12

You can acquire **emotional control** by taking these evidence-based, concrete measures:

Calm down and identify your feelings.

Here are several methods to break up heightened emotions:

- Recognize your physical cues: Being triggered is indicated by shortness of breath, an elevated heart rate, a louder voice, and sweating.
- Make a strategy for how you will pause and regain your balance.
- Wash your face and hands.
- Go outside to get some fresh air.
- Listen to music.

The goal is to give yourself some breathing room between how you feel and what you want to accomplish. You could try the following techniques to do that:

- Note down the plans on your phone to easily access them.

- You can take a break when someone or something is bothering you.
- You could also try saying, "Let us take a break for ten minutes, and then we will continue this conversation."

Practice mindfulness

Recent studies show mindfulness can help children and adults with ADHD symptoms (Honos-Webb, 2011). Consider trying one or all of these three meditation methods:

- Sitting meditation
- Body scan
- Meditative yoga

Being mindful of your body helps you return to the present moment. This awareness might provide you with the necessary break to redirect strong emotions. It can also help in the development of emotional awareness. You can participate in mindfulness activities through churches, community centers, or online. Many applications let you practice mindfulness in your own home.

Pay attention to your thoughts and take notes.

According to a comparative research study, women with ADHD often unintentionally indulge in the following thought patterns (Mitchell et al., 2013):

- Self-blame: "It is my fault."
- Accusing others: "They should not have done that."
- Catastrophizing: "This is the worst thing ever."
- Reflecting: "If only, what if...."

Consider putting your ideas down on paper if you are feeling sad. It may take some effort, but you can try evaluating recurring negative thoughts:

- I accomplished one thing correctly.
- They may have had good reasons for what they did.
- Despite the difficult start to the day, things are improving.
- I will let it go for the time being and try again tomorrow.

Bodywork

Emotional regulation and ADHD are both influenced by your mind and your body. According to a research analysis of ADHD, adults and children can benefit from exercise (Mitchell et al., 2013).

- Executive function and emotional control are enhanced by exercise.
- Exercise that involves cardio is incredibly beneficial.

- Non-cardio exercise has an impact as well.

Journal Your Way to a Happier Self

ADHD journeys can become more enjoyable through writing. Writing is an excellent way to:

- Clarify your thoughts and emotions.
- Learn more about yourself.
- Reduce tension. It helps to reduce the intensity of painful emotions like grief, rage, and pain by writing about them. You feel more at ease and are more adept at staying in the present.
- More efficiently resolving issues. We often approach problem-solving from an analytical, left-brained perspective. Engaging the right brain's instincts may lead to a better solution. This part of the brain is made accessible by writing, which opens the door to creative solutions.
- Resolve conflicts with others. Writing about communication issues rather than dwelling on them encourages you to consider other perspectives. You are more likely to resolve the conflict reasonably.

Rejection! What Is It and How Can I Deal With It?

Even though there is no official diagnosis or disorder for rejection sensitivity, many women claim that the most detrimental aspect of their ADHD is their inability to manage their emotions to rejection. Anxiety, stress, guilt, and rejection impact their quality of life.

Although some susceptible women detect rejection in superficial interactions, the most traumatic incidents involve rejection from close ones. Recovering from a painful exchange might take hours.

Society encourages women to fulfill their social obligations to meet the needs of others. Although girls with ADHD encounter this obligation early on, they discover that their brains are not built to be sensitive to the emotions of others.

For being highly sensitive, often confused, and unable to pick up on social cues, they are often bullied and rejected by their peers. Many girls with ADHD exhibit behaviours that irritate others, making them easy targets for criticism. Their ingrained fear of rejection mirrors their inability to adapt to social norms.

Excessive stress drives the brain to respond in powerful ways, even at the cost of compromising other functions. Many women with ADHD were subjected to chronic negative criticism as children, including severe punishment, bullying, rejection, and humiliation from family, friends, and teachers. Women with ADHD feel like impostors after decades of rejection, afraid that their perceived failures would be exposed and trigger rejection.

◆ ◆ ◆

Date ---------

Exercise 13

Women with ADHD regularly experience rejection sensitivity dysphoria (RSD), or the intense emotional suffering related to emotions of rejection and shame. Take this self-test to check whether your symptoms are similar to RSD.

Rating scale:

- 1= Never
- 2= Rarely
- 3= Sometimes
- 4= Often
- 5= Very Often

Questionnaire:

1. Do you have fits of ager when your feelings are hurt?

   1 2 3 4

2. Do you ever experience extreme sadness when you think you have been rejected or criticized?

   1 2 3 4

3. Are you your own worst critic?

1 2 3 4

4. Do you have anxiety in social situations because you feel no one likes you?

   1 2 3 4

5. Are you a people pleaser?

   1 2 3 4

6. Do you turn down opportunities or delay starting tasks because you fear failing?

   1 2 3 4

7. Because of your intense emotional responses, have you ever been considered overly sensitive?

   1 2 3 4

8. Do you spend more time working on a project than is required?

   1 2 3 4

9. Do you ever feel your emotions physically, as if you have been hit in the chest or somehow injured?

   1 2 3 4

10. Are you ashamed of your "lack of control" over your emotions?

    1 2 3 4

11. Were you told you had a personality disorder before you were diagnosed with ADHD?

    1 2 3 4

12. Do you avoid deep friendships or

romantic connections out of fear that others will not like you when they get to know you?

1 2 3 4

13. Do you always expect the worst in everyday interactions?

    1 2 3 4

14. Do you think you cannot continue to feel this way?

    1 2 3 4

15. Do you avoid exploring new things or meeting new people because you fear rejection and criticism?

    1 2 3 4

You can use this questionnaire to see if you have symptoms of rejection sensitivity distress (RSD). If the majority of the questions were answered with "Often" or "Very Often," you should find a qualified mental health professional since it is possible that you could be going through signs of rejection-sensitive dysphoria. Only a clinical assessment can lead to an accurate diagnosis.

Understanding and Managing Your Emotional Triggers

You go through various feelings every day, including excitement, anxiety, anger, pleasure, and disappointment. These are often linked to specific situations, such as job interviews, conversations with friends, or interactions with your partner. Your reaction to these experiences will differ depending on your state of mind and the variables that affect the situation.

Any memory, experience, or incident that causes a strong emotional response, regardless of how you feel, is an emotional trigger. Good emotional health mainly depends on being aware of your emotional triggers and knowing how to manage them.
Everyone has emotional triggers, although they may differ from person to person. Painful memories, uncomfortable subjects, someone else's words or actions, or even your behaviours could all be triggered. Situations that usually cause strong emotions to arise include:

- Rejection
- Betrayal
- Unequal treatment
- Contradictory ideologies
- Becoming helpless or losing control
- Being left out or neglected
- Criticism
- Being unwanted or disliked
- Feeling suffocated or needy, insecurity
- Loss of autonomy

◆ ◆ ◆

Date --------

Exercise 14

In order to identify your emotional triggers, you have to:

- **Be aware of your body and mind.** Paying attention to when circumstances cause a strong emotional response is an essential first step in learning to identify your triggers. In addition to heightened emotions, anxiety can also manifest physically as a racing heart, stomach ache, dizziness or trembling, and moist palms.

- **Step back.** When you see these signs, pause to reflect on what just happened and the reaction it triggered. Imagine you spend the entire day re-organizing and cleaning your house. You excitedly wait for your partner's response when they leave work. Instead, they walk into the bathroom without saying anything. Because your efforts went unnoticed, you are upset, frustrated, and angry. You feel your heart racing and your jaw clenched. It takes all your willpower to resist snapping and saying something you will regret later.

- **Track the origins.** Try tracing the source of these emotions by recalling previous experiences that gave rise to the feelings you are currently experiencing. Perhaps it suddenly seemed like you were a teenager once again, striving to keep the house spotless to win the approval of an absent parent. When the emotional trigger is activated, you are instantly taken back to that moment when you believed that nothing you did was worthwhile.

- **Get curious.** It would help to dig deeper because the link can be more complex. Do not try to ignore or fight off intense emotions as they arise. Instead, please address them to learn more about what could have caused them. Are there any patterns? Career discussions, for example, might evoke feelings of resentment and frustration associated with your fear of underachievement.

You might think that all you need to do to manage your emotions is to avoid the circumstances that set them off. However, it is more complicated. There are some tricky situations in life that you cannot prevent or get out of, and those uncomfortable feelings are bound to come back.

Here are some ideas to help you in managing them at the moment:

- **Own your emotions.** Begin by reminding yourself that whatever emotion you are experiencing at the time is perfectly normal. It is usual for triggers to evoke a wide range of feelings, including sadness, anger, and fear. However, it would be best to embrace those feelings before you can deal with them. Over time, it only gets worse if you suppress or deny how you are feeling.

It might be helpful to remind yourself of the differences between the past and the present, but do it with compassion for yourself rather than judgment. You can feel stressed and frustrated about a particular situation and wish to respond a certain way. Instead, accept that while past incidents may have hurt you, they are not the same now. This might help you in regaining control and carefully choose another response.

- **Take a break for a while.** You can prevent emotional overload by withdrawing physically. Excuse yourself if you need a moment to yourself. This can help you avoid a reflex response you might regret later. Do some breathing or grounding exercises to relax and calm yourself. The goal here is not to prevent situations that trigger certain emotions altogether. Just give yourself a moment to cool down to help you respond to the problem more effectively. You may return to the situation with more clarity once you have calmed down.

- **Keep an open mind.** Most people do not intentionally try to make you feel miserable. Some of their acts or comments that bother you may result from their emotional triggers or other reasons you are unaware of. When your partner arrived, didn't they notice you had cleaned the entire house? They might have had a difficult day, received terrible news, and needed time to recover before discussing it. You might only be aware of the emotions that someone is experiencing once they express them to you. Misjudging their actions or intentions is easier when you do not know someone well. This underlines how important it is to take their perspective into account.

- **Communicate.** When someone's behaviour triggers your emotions, speaking out may help you avoid a similar occurrence. Take a moment to regain your composure and try addressing the issue with statements that begin with "I" to communicate constructively. Instead of hurling things around and shouting, "Where did you put my book?" Try saying, "I get frustrated when you take my things without asking and do not return them." It could be helpful in some situations to encourage the other person to communicate more effectively. Try asking someone politely, "What is on your mind?" if they are being silent, acting passive-aggressively, or making harsh or sarcastic remarks.

How to Get Over Insecurity and Improve Self-Esteem

It is common to have bad days when you feel good for nothing. However, constant self-doubt may negatively impact all aspects of your life, including your physical health, emotional stability, and work performance. Low self-esteem makes you more prone to jealousy and anxiety, which can be very dangerous for your relationships.

The good news is that you can improve your sense of self-esteem. Even though it will not happen immediately, you can gradually change your feelings about yourself with the correct strategies and attitude.

◆ ◆ ◆

Date ---------

Exercise 15

Things to do:

- **Establish your value.** Make a list of all the things you are doing well. The hundreds of positive micro-decisions you make daily probably need to be considered in your ideas about yourself. Focusing on your accomplishments rather than your flaws might be achieved by remembering how you helped your neighbour carry their bags.

- **Prioritize attending to your needs.** You must treat yourself properly if you always attend to everyone else's needs while overlooking your own. You may fight negative thoughts and boost your self-worth by adding self-care into your daily routine.

- **Embrace awkwardness.** You will stumble occasionally; it is just a fact of life. However, acknowledging this reality might make you more at ease in your skin. Try to laugh it off the next time you experience embarrassment or self-consciousness.

- **Confront your negative thinking.** When we stumble or make a mistake, it is easy to be hard on ourselves. However, beating yourself up because you did not get the big promotion or failed a test leaves you trapped in a vicious cycle of guilt and self-hatred. Try to get in the habit of challenging your negative thoughts as they arise. Forgive yourself, and recognize that these are isolated incidents that do not represent you as a person. If you have negative thoughts, write them down so you can stand aside and observe them. Refocus on the positives after considering what you have gained from experience. You can use what you have learned to improve future outcomes.

- **Spend time with your loved ones.** There is no better way to boost your self-esteem and feel accepted for who you are than to surround yourself with loving, supportive people. Plan to meet up with your loved ones more often. It will be easier for you to appreciate your unique qualities if you can see yourself through the eyes of others who love you.

- **Stay away from unpleasant circumstances.** You may narrow down who and what to avoid by identifying the people and situations undermining your self-esteem. Finding a better company should be your priority if you are surrounded by people who constantly criticize you.

- **Think of the positives.** When you have accomplished a remarkable milestone at work, celebrate it and congratulate yourself. Even though it feels strange at first, being proud of what you do may significantly impact your self-esteem. Please write down your successes so you may return to them when feeling insecure. You can also take a few minutes each day to list three positive features of yourself. This will serve as a reminder to help you feel more confident throughout the day.

- **Do things that make you happy.** Spend your leisure time doing activities that make you happy and satisfied, whether reading a book or preparing a delicious dinner. Consider picking up a hobby you have always wanted to pursue, or even better, learn a new skill. Learning a new skill makes you happy and reminds you of your abilities and interests.

- **Aim for baby steps.** It takes time to overcome insecurity and boost your self-esteem. Try to be patient with yourself during this process, and keep going even if things do not get better as quickly as you would like them to. Even if you do not feel secure right now, keep pushing forward because your small baby steps will ultimately blossom into larger ones.

- **Work with a therapist.** Talking with a qualified therapist can help you understand the source of your anxieties and insecurities. They can also assist you in creating new strategies for dealing with circumstances that make you feel insecure.

- **Read the books.** Books that discuss the causes of insecurity and strategies for overcoming it might provide helpful information and make you feel less isolated in your struggles.

Sky Rocketing My Self Esteem!

Studies show that self-esteem increases consistently over time and peaks at age 60. This generalization does not apply to everyone with ADHD, for whom self-esteem and confidence keep falling as they age. Many older women feel underwhelmed and frustrated and perceive themselves as a failure when it comes to their peers. Many people feel hopeless after years of unsuccessful behaviour modification efforts.

The good news is that as they age, women with ADHD can rebuild their self-confidence and self-esteem. It involves managing ADHD as effectively as possible and preventing negative thoughts.

◆◆◆

Date ---------

Exercise 16

Even though negative thoughts appear natural, they cannot be considered typical or healthy. Instead, consider these thoughts to be cognitive illusions. Although the battle for a better self will be lengthy, it can be won.

Here are 11 strategies for overcoming negative thoughts and regaining self-confidence:

1. Recognize and accept your ADHD, then concentrate on changing your behaviour.
2. ADHD is not a personality flaw. It is a set of manageable neurobiological symptoms.
3. It is never too late to develop improved ADHD management skills. Avoid using the justification "I have tried everything."
4. Recognize and value your achievements.
5. Evaluate your strengths and weaknesses. If this is difficult, seek outside advice.
6. Identify, observe, analyze, and dismiss your critical self-talk. With practice and patience, the battle will become easier over time.
7. Avoid comparing yourself to others.

8. Pay attention to solutions, not problems. "What can I do about it?" should be your next thought after identifying a problem.
9. Ignore what you have yet to accomplish in the past. Pay attention to the task at hand.
10. Look for supportive connections. Spend time with those that respect and understand who you are.
11. Look after your body well. Sleep, exercise, and food all significantly affect your mood.

Let's Build a Plan to Regain Confidence

Sometimes people set themselves up for failure by setting overly broad, unreasonable, or unreachable goals. Consider setting a goal like, "I want to be more confident." There needs to be a clear action plan for achieving this goal, which lacks direction and specificity. As there is no guidance on what you want to do, how to accomplish it, or when to do it, you end up forgetting about them over time.

However, when you set SMART goals, you avoid a negative outcome since your SMART goal is clearly stated. With such clarity of concept, you are more likely to focus on your goal, which will help you achieve it.

Some examples of SMART Goals for increasing confidence:

1. Improve eye contact.
2. Improve listening skills.
3. Correct my posture.
4. Avoid using too many filler words.
5. Public speaking practice.
6. Speak up more often.
7. Extend my network
8. Improve time management skills.

Date ---------

Exercise 17

Goal 1: Improve eye contact

The elements of SMART goal:

- Specific: Improve your eye contact with at least five individuals.
- Measurable: By tracking how long you maintained eye contact, you can determine whether you are progressing toward your goal.
- Achievable: You can accomplish this goal since numerous people with low confidence have already attained it.
- Relevant: Making eye contact better is a critical component of boosting confidence.
- Time-Bound: The timeline is set at thirty days of practice.

Complete SMART goal: I want to improve my eye contact with everyone I meet to boost my credibility. I will accomplish this by maintaining extended eye contact for more than five seconds or longer with at least five people I meet over the next 30 days.

Goal 2: Improve listening skills

The elements of SMART goal:

- Specific: You want to be a good listener who is impartial and open-minded.
- Measurable: You can count the people you encounter each day as a measure.
- Achievable: The goal is achievable for those who have done it before.
- Relevant: Improving your listening skills is essential to having confidence.
- Time-Bound: You have given yourself a thirty-day window to form new habits.

Complete SMART goal:

During the next thirty days, I will intentionally listen effectively to everyone I encounter. I want to be a responsive and nonjudgmental listener.

Secondly, put a challenge on yourself to establish concrete goals that you strive toward every day. Creating SMART goals for confidence is essential because it enables you to focus on a vague goal and convert it into concrete methods you can apply to feel more at ease throughout your life. Start by selecting a couple of the SMART goals for confidence from the provided list to get the most out of your goal-setting efforts.

◆ ◆ ◆

Key Takeaways

- Women with ADHD struggle with emotional regulation and are more sensitive to rejection due to how their brains process information and stimuli.

- Understanding your emotional triggers and how to respond to them can help you manage your emotions and reduce stress.

- Self-reflection and mindfulness practices, like meditation, can help increase self-awareness and promote emotional stability.

- Building self-esteem through positive self-talk and engaging in activities that bring a sense of accomplishment can help women with ADHD handle rejection and criticism better.

- Seeking support from loved ones, therapists, or support groups can help women with ADHD cope with the emotional challenges of living with the disorder.

- Learning effective communication strategies and conflict-resolution techniques can improve relationships and reduce stress.

After exploring the relationship between ADHD

and emotions, it is time to move on to another area of life that can be challenging for those with ADHD–keeping the home organized. If you are tired of living in clutter and want to learn how to create a more organized and stress-free environment, the next chapter, "How to Declutter My Home and Keep it Organized," is for you.

This chapter offers practical tips and strategies for decluttering your home and maintaining a tidy space, including how to get started, what to do with sentimental items, and how to stay organized over the long term. Do not let a messy home hold you back–take the first step toward creating a more peaceful and organized living space by reading the next chapter.

◆ ◆ ◆

CHAPTER 5: HOW TO DECLUTTER MY HOME AND KEEP IT ORGANIZED?

Clutter can be a source of stress and anxiety for individuals with ADHD, making it all the more important to prioritize decluttering as a self-care practice. –Dr. Michele Novotni.

Living with ADHD can make it challenging to stay on top of everyday tasks, including keeping your home clean and organized. However, clutter and disorganization can exacerbate ADHD symptoms, leading to feelings of overwhelm and stressed.

This chapter will explore practical strategies for

decluttering your home and creating an organized space that supports your mental health. From simple organization hacks to daily routines that keep your home in order, you will learn how to make your living space a haven of peace and productivity. You can also refer to my best-selling books *Decluttering Your Home In A Year Or Less!* and *Organize Your Home In A Year Or Less* for more detailed advice and complete plan and worksheets to declutter and organize your home.

It is healthy for you to maintain a clean home and keep it clutter-free. Studies show that cleanliness, or the lack of it, can directly affect mental health. Compared to women who claimed their houses were relaxing and regenerative, those who said their homes were cluttered or overflowing with unfinished chores were more likely to feel worn out and depressed.

Clutter symbolizes unfinished business to the brain, and for some people, this can be highly distressing. Clutter can lead to increased tension and anxiety. Since clutter is associated with negative emotions like confusion, anxiety, and irritability, it can be challenging to concentrate on a specific task. Still, by cleaning, organizing, and decluttering, people can take control of their surroundings and create a more relaxing environment that helps them focus on other important matters.

Decluttering can improve your mental health in many ways. For example, it gives you a sense of control over your surroundings. It involves your mind in a repetitive task that can be relaxing. Also, it has been proven to elevate mood and provide a sense of satisfaction. Decluttering can relieve stress for several reasons.

Some advantages of decluttering and organizing your home or office are:

- **Cleaning has health benefits.** A tidy house influences your physical well-being. Research has found that people who live in clean homes are often healthier than those who live in disorganized or cluttered homes (Matlen, 2020).

- **Take charge of your environment.** Cleaning can be a way for people to regain some control over their lives. Concentrating or finishing other tasks can be difficult because of the distractions caused by clutter and disorder, which might make you feel trapped. Therefore, if you feel the impulse to clean and organize your living space when you are anxious or stressed, your mind and body are probably trying to find a way to create order in your surroundings.

- **Enhance your mood.** Besides the obvious benefits of having a cleaner home, the relationship between cleanliness and mental health can help minimize anxiety. For example, people who were mindful while doing chores claim to be far less anxious and more inspired. According to studies, making your bed and having clean sheets are related to a good night's sleep (Matlen, 2020). A proper sleeping routine provides many mental health benefits, including an improved mood. Cleaning can also help to reduce depressive symptoms and fatigue and increase attention.

- **Improve your concentration.** You may find concentrating difficult when your home needs to be more organized, organized, or extremely dirty. Also, the clutter makes it harder for your brain to process information. Try cleaning your workspace first if you have problems concentrating on a task. Setting aside only a few minutes to arrange your possessions and tidy up any clutter can help you focus and accomplish your task more quickly. Minimizing your belongings can have the same effect since it limits the number of things competing for your brain's attention.

ADHD and Space Organization

Despite how absurd it may sound, disorganization can wreck your life. Disorganization is perhaps most noticeable in women with ADHD. They need help planning things out and struggle to manage their time, thoughts, and information. People with ADHD tend to organize by creating piles that, over time, grow like weeds. You need to create structure in your everyday life to compensate for what is lacking inside your mind.

Time management skills can be developed by observing the passing of time. The structure can be anything, an alarm clock, a key chain, or even a basket to keep the keys when you return home.

You can also pre-set alarms to remind yourself to complete chores or when to take daily medication. Each time you sit down to study or work on a project, start by setting the timer for 20 minutes. After a 5-minute rest, continue for another 20. You can use Post-It Notes to remind yourself of the number of tasks. Initiating and utilizing these tools takes time and practice, so setting them up provides a necessary structure.

It is not necessary for women with ADHD to become extremely tidy freaks; this is often beyond their capacity. They only need to organize themselves effectively to accomplish their goals. Some essential tools for organizing are:

- Creating a list
- Keeping anything important in one place that is easy to find
- Using flashcards and other memory aids to help remember important information
- Finding things quickly.

Five W's of Setting Goals

Being organized takes effort. Expecting to become fully organized this month if you have not been in the past few months or years is unrealistic. Setting small weekly goals for organizing your house will make the process easier. It will give you more time to complete other daily chores and allow you to celebrate little triumphs.

Keep a diary or journal to keep track of your progress, inspirations, setbacks, and emotions. Take a moment to reflect on the positives of being organized and how that will make you feel. Consider the five W's while making goals:

- **Why** is it essential for you to get organized?
- **Where** do you need structure the most?
- **When** will you accomplish your goals?
- **Who** will benefit from the organization?
- **What** do you intend to organize?

Set Realistic Organizing Goals

Setting goals is the first step toward accomplishing anything. Write down specific goals rather than vague ones like "organize my house" since you need to know your aim. It has to be broken down into more realistic and specific goals. Create multiple, smaller goals.

You will soon be able to take a step back and see how each action brought you one step closer to obtaining an organized house. Please write down your goals and check them off as you complete them. Make your goals as detailed as necessary to experience the thrill of accomplishment as you check them off your list.

◆ ◆ ◆

Date ---------

Exercise 18

Step 1: Get rid of useless things

The first thing to do is go through each room and remove stuff as much as possible. You only want to organize what you intend to keep, which will also help streamline your task. Any damaged goods, something you can no longer use, expired items, and anything too dirty to use should be thrown away. Make another box of things to donate once you have disposed of the damaged things. These should be things that are in excellent shape but rarely used. You might need to spend an entire weekend on this process, but push until you have nothing except things you genuinely love and intend to use.

Step 2: Start small by organizing drawers

Once you have gotten rid of anything you do not need, it is time to organize what you did keep. Set a goal of organizing every drawer in your house. You can buy some handy drawer organizers online. While it could take some time, you will feel great after organizing each drawer.

Step 3: Make room for your things

☐ Make space for all of your belongings. Just move from room to room and list everything you need to create a place. Write down all that has been left out and requires a basket, bag, or donation. Places where clutter often develops include:

- ☐ Above the refrigerator
- ☐ Breakfast bar or kitchen island
- ☐ The sink counters
- ☐ The space near the doorway

Step 4: Organize closet space

Organizing all of your closets should be your next priority. This applies to all closets, including those in bedrooms, bathrooms, and even the garage. Once you are done, you will realize that you do not need to spend much time looking for what you need from the closet, and everything is right there.

Step 5: Organize the cabinets

Browse the kitchen and bathroom cabinets to find the proper setup for you and your family. After organizing the closets, arrange the cabinets. Try out different arrangements till you find the ideal one for you. Stay calm if it takes a while.

Step 6: Get your family onboard

Everyone living in the house should keep it organized. Whether your partner works too much or your children are too young to contribute, you can still have their support. Ask them to help you by maintaining the system that you have created.

Step 7: Set a purpose for each room

What function does the living room serve? How about your workplace? Addressing this question will help you develop organizational methods and keep unnecessary objects out of those spaces. There should not be toys all over your workspace. Establish separate zones if you live in a compact space where your living room serves numerous purposes. Consider dividing one corner as the play area, where the toys belong, and the other as the entertainment section, to keep the video games and gaming consoles.

Step 8: Organize one room at a time

Lastly, attending to just one room at a time is essential. Organize one closet or drawer at a time. It is so easy to become overwhelmed and give up. Remember, it is not necessary to do everything in one go. Establish achievable goals to spare yourself the stress.

Declutter Your Home

You do not even realize how, little by bit, you bring things into your home. Eventually, they begin to weigh on you, suffocating you until you are so overwhelmed that you cannot breathe. To declutter your house, grab a trash bag and go through the list below as you move from room to room.

◆ ◆ ◆

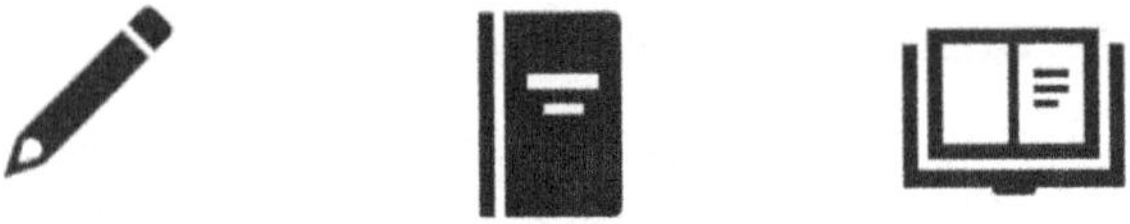

Date ---------

Exercise 19

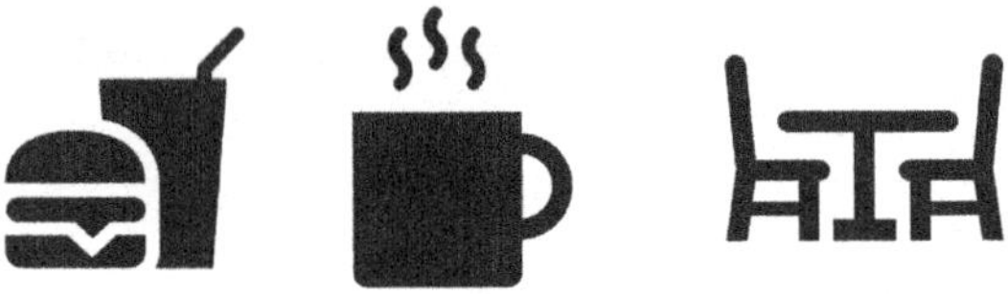

Kitchen

- ☐ Throw out outdated spices.
- ☐ Throw away any expired food from the pantry and cabinets.
- ☐ Sell or donate extra baking supplies.
- ☐ Sell or donate kitchenware that you last used over a year ago.
- ☐ Throw away dishes that are broken or chipped.
- ☐ Sell or donate old or unused table settings.
- ☐ Replace the kitchen sponge.
- ☐ Recycle plastic and paper bags.
- ☐ Donate the mugs you last used a long time ago.

- [ ] Sort the papers on the counter.
- [ ] Recycle your garbage.
- [ ] Clear out the junk drawer.

Living room

☐ The garbage under the couch cushions.

☐ Everything from under the couch.

☐ Sell or donate the pillows that are usually on the floor.

☐ Give away or sell the children's chairs that nobody
uses anymore.

Bathroom

- [ ] Get rid of the shampoo bottles and hotel soaps from your trip two years ago.
- [ ] Get rid of expired makeup products.
- [ ] Throw away old toothbrushes.
- [ ] Throw away expired medicines.
- [ ] Get rid of the toilet brush.
- [ ] Discard the stack of used tissue boxes and empty toilet paper rolls.
- [ ] Throw away expired sunscreen.
- [ ] Get rid of the clutter in the drawer.
- [ ] Throw away dirty and worn-out washcloths and towels.

Office

☐ Throw away outdated receipts.

☐ Go through the stack of mail you have never opened.

☐ Recycle old catalogues and magazines.

☐ Throw away damaged crayons, empty markers, and
pens that do not work.

☐ Throw out any cables that you need to know where
they go.

☐ Unless you are planning to use the half-used note
books, recycle them.

☐ Recycle the office supplies you have owned for years.

☐ Sort through the piles of documents in the drawers.

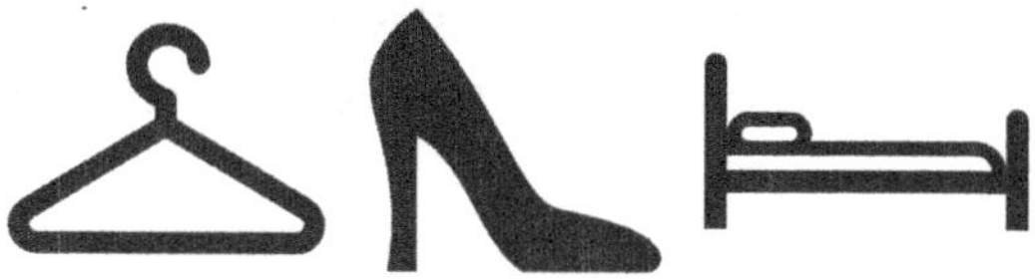

Bedroom

- [ ] Go through your wardrobe.
- [ ] Donate or sell clothes that do not fit well or that you have not worn in a year.
- [ ] Look through your underwear drawer and throw away anything torn or no longer fits.
- [ ] Toss the socks that are still missing their matching.
- [ ] Throw away faded and old clothes.
- [ ] Sort and donate the pile of books near the bedside table.
- [ ] Give away any old or uncomfortable shoes you no longer wear.
- [ ] Sift your jewelry, and donate the old items you do not use anymore.

☐ Sort the bags and purses.
☐ Clear out the contents of the dresser drawer.

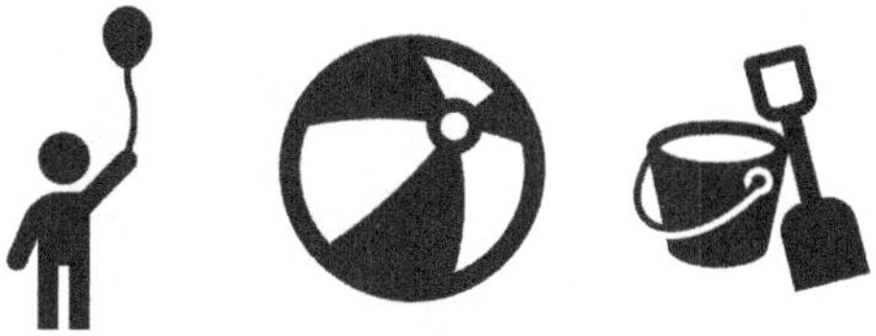

Playroom

- [ ] Throw away damaged toys.
- [ ] Sell or donate duplicate toys.
- [ ] Donate or sell your children's old toys that are still in good shape.
- [ ] Give away or sell the toys your kids no longer play with or are too old for.
- [ ] Throw away puzzles and board games that have missing pieces.
- [ ] Sort through the craft supplies. Toss any broken crayons and dried-up markers.

Rest of the house

- ☐ Please remember to replace the smoke detector batter
  ies after recycling them.
- ☐ Donate or sell any furniture that does not fit in the
  room.
- ☐ Make a list as you move from room to room.
- ☐ Sell or donate home decor that no longer matches
  your home or aesthetic.
- ☐ Recycle old cell phones.
- ☐ Recycle old laptops and computers.
- ☐ Check the vacuum filter.
- ☐ Replace the air filters.

Create a Chore List and a Reward List

Making a chore list that specifies everyone's roles is an excellent way to involve the entire family. This will not only ease the stress on the person who usually handles things around the house, but it will also reduce tension in the house and maintain family bonding time.

What you choose to include on your chore list should be based on four factors:

1. Things you must complete.

2. Things you want to be consistent at.

3. Things that improve your health.

4. Things you usually need to remember to do.

Date ---------

Exercise 20

By creating your chore list, you can ensure that no chores are missed and that each day of the week has a reasonable number of tasks assigned. Make a list of all the tasks that must be completed first, and then include the names of the family members in charge of each task.

The following is an example of the chore list:

- ☐ Washing dishes every day
- ☐ Putting away the dishes after drying them
- ☐ Mopping and sweeping
- ☐ Vacuuming the carpets dusting
- ☐ Doing laundry
- ☐ Watering the plants
- ☐ Daily pet feedings
- ☐ Each family member makes their bed and cleans up their room
- ☐ Raking leaves, trimming the grass, and removing weeds

The list has to be created specifically for your family's requirements.

The following is an example of the reward list:

- Cash
- Coffee
- Gift cards
- Dinner
- Movie
- Car wash
- Manicure and pedicure
- New purse
- New shoes
- New gadget
- New book
- Expensive wine
- Road trip
- A class for learning a new skill
- Online subscriptions
- New tool

◆ ◆ ◆

Key Takeaways

- Women with ADHD struggle with organization and clutter due to how their brains process information and manage tasks.
- Breaking down decluttering and organizing tasks into smaller, manageable steps can make the process less daunting and more achievable.
- Developing a routine or schedule for cleaning and organizing can help make it a consistent habit, which may be more effective than sporadic or occasional bursts of effort.
- Limiting the amount of stuff you have helps to keep your home organized and clutter-free.
- Celebrating your successes and recognizing your progress can help you stay motivated and build momentum to keep your home organized.

The next chapter, "How to Manage My Relationships With ADHD?" provides practical tools and strategies to navigate the challenges of maintaining healthy and fulfilling relationships. You will learn about the common issues people with ADHD face in their relationships and tips for effective communication, setting boundaries, and managing conflict. So do not wait; read on and take control of your relationships today!

◆ ◆ ◆

CHAPTER 6: HOW TO MANAGE MY RELATIONSHIPS WITH ADHD?

ADHD can impact not only romantic relationships but also friendships and family dynamics. –Dr. Roberto Olivardia.

Living with ADHD can impact all areas of your life, including your relationships with others. Whether with romantic partners, family members, or friends, this disorder can create unique challenges in maintaining healthy, fulfilling connections with others.

This chapter will explore practical strategies for managing your relationships with ADHD, from effective communication and boundary-setting to cultivating empathy and building a support network. You will learn how to navigate common challenges that can arise in relationships with ADHD and develop the skills to create strong, supportive connections with the people who matter most.

Avoid Isolation, Get Out of the Dead-Zone

For women with ADHD, social isolation is a serious problem. When family members and coworkers do not understand their struggles with ADHD, they feel cut off from them. Moreover, they feel too ashamed to even ask for help. Although social relationships are something that both sexes can struggle with, there is often a double standard.

While a man may get away with breaking one of the many societal rules, a woman usually does not, even if it is the same rule. The reason is that women are expected to be more knowledgeable about appropriate social behaviours.

Many women with ADHD feel their social skills are lacking in the following areas:

- Feeling socially connected with friends, acquaintances, and business partners.
- Being able to switch between work, home, and family.

- Being able to ask for help or assert needs.

As a result, they feel lonely and depressed due to a lack of good social connections.

◆ ◆ ◆

Date --------

Exercise 21

- **Connect with friends.** Social skills include everything we should and should not say or do while interacting with others. We are all expected to know the social norms that control our interactions and relationships. Without feedback, it is not easy to improve your social behaviour. You often get dismissed, rejected, and lonely without understanding what you did wrong. No one usually tells you, either.

What to do: Get advice from people you can trust to help you identify the social skill areas where you need improvement and be open to criticism. You can get help from others with your blind spots.

At-home guidance: Take a social skills test to identify your strengths and weaknesses.

- **Multi-tasking.** Men usually have the luxury of focusing on one thing at a time. However, that is only sometimes the case with women, especially given their societal expectations that they will run the household and serve as social organizers. They manage household duties, while multi-tasking can cause severe problems for those with ADHD. Many women feel exhausted and low in self-esteem if they fail to carry out these everyday activities. The amount of physical and mental exhaustion makes it difficult to focus on social interactions. To prevent embarrassment, many women avoid social situations.

What to do: If disorganization is getting in your social life, consider seeking guidance from a coach to help you build effective methods, structure, and support to remove this block.

At-home guidance: Let go of the notion that women must "be everything to everyone" and be able to "do it all" for their partners and families. Your younger children can fold clothes or pick things up off the floor, your older children may enjoy making dinner or packing lunches for school, and your partner can pick up groceries on his way home.

- **Assert yourself.** Unsurprisingly, women often find it difficult to express their wants and needs. Despite their desire for change, many women hesitate to ask for it or take risks. This usually creates a gap in social interactions and interpersonal communication.

What to do: Try taking an assertiveness training class. Counselling offices offer these courses to help you communicate your needs and want more clearly and effectively.

At-home guidance:

1. If uncomfortable making big requests, start small and work your way up.
2. Ask your partner to get the groceries.
3. Ask a friend to join you for lunch at your choice of restaurant.

Taking the lead reduces anxiety about how a situation will turn out.

- **Manage your ADHD feelings**. Women are often more socially conscious than men, making them more aware of their isolation or inability to meet social standards. This often results in loneliness and mood disorders.

What to do: If you have trouble identifying and expressing your feelings, you probably struggle with your self-esteem or mood. Consider the possible benefits of therapy to help you have a better social life.

At-home guidance: Join one of the many forums, chat rooms, or support groups for women dealing with ADHD and discover that you are not alone.

You can develop social skills that will improve how you interact with people. Try to improve your social skills and nurture the relationships that might make you feel connected.

Am I a Good Friend?

We often overlook the importance of friendship quality. We make acquaintances as we move through life, and we meet them at work, school, or through a friend. Some of those acquaintances become friends, and a few of those friends join our inner circle. We do not take a moment to consider whether these friends are the right people to spend our time with or whether we are good friends to them.

Date ---------

Exercise 22

Use this reflection exercise to stand back and evaluate the quality of your most important friendships. Rank your top ten friends based on the following criteria:

- Best friend
- Perfect friend
- Good friend

Do you believe that your friends would place you in the same categories as you have? If not, then why? How do you think that impacts the nature of your friendship daily?

Ten questions to ask yourself

1. How much time do you spend with that friend each week?

   ----

2. How would you rate the overall quality of that timespan?

3. What qualities do you admire about your friend?

4. Is your friendship drama-free?

5. What is it about your friend that you do not like?

6. If you could, what would you change about your friendship?

7. In terms of giving and receiving, is the friendship balanced?

8. What could you do to improve your friendship with them?

9. Which of your memories of your friend is your favorite?

10. Do you feel happy both during and after socializing with them?

Try repeating this exercise for your "excellent" and "good" friends. By reflecting on your friendships, you might realize that you should put more effort into one or need to have a difficult conversation with a friend. You may recognize that a friend you once considered your best friend is not someone you should keep in your close circle.

Be a Popular Person!

Having ADHD does not mean that you cannot be a famous person. It is essential to focus on your strengths and interests to become more popular and find social activities that align with them. You could join a club or group related to your interests, such as a sports team or a music club. Additionally, try to be positive and friendly toward others and take the time to listen to them when they speak.

Engage in conversations by asking questions and showing interest in what they say. Finally, try to be open about your ADHD and share your experiences with others. This can help people understand and appreciate your unique perspective and may even encourage others with ADHD to connect with you.

Remember, being famous is not about changing who you are but embracing your strengths and finding ways to connect with others who share your interests and passions. Answering these questions will help you take the first step toward becoming popular:

Date ---------

Exercise 23

Self-acceptance:

1. How can self-acceptance help me be more confident and less self-conscious?

2. What are some ways to practice self-compassion and self-love?

3. What are some strategies to overcome negative self-talk and self-criticism?

4. How can I balance self-improvement with self-acceptance?

5. What role do mindfulness and meditation play in promoting self-acceptance?

Using technology for building new friendships:

1. What online platforms or apps can help me meet new people?

2. How can I use social media to expand my network and make new friends?

3. What common pitfalls to avoid when using technology to make new friends?

4. How can I stay safe when using online platforms to meet new people?

5. How can I transition from online communication to in-person meetings with new friends?

Being comfortable talking about your ADHD:

1. How can I educate myself about ADHD to feel more comfortable talking about it?

2. What are some strategies to manage ADHD symptoms in social situations?

3. How can I help others understand the impact of ADHD on my daily life?

4. What are some ways to advocate for ADHD accommodations at school or work?

5. How can I connect with others with ADHD to build a support network?

Understanding triggers:

1. How can I track my triggers to understand my emotional reactions better?

2. What are some coping strategies to manage triggers at the moment?

3. How can I develop a personalized self-care plan to reduce triggers?

4. What are some techniques for addressing past trauma that may be triggering?

5. How can therapy help me identify and manage triggers?

Activities you like most:

1. What are your favourite hobbies or activities, and why do you enjoy them?

2. How can you incorporate your favourite activities into your daily routine?

3. How can you use your interests to connect with others who share similar passions?

4. What are some new activities you would like to try, and why?

5. How can you challenge yourself to push beyond your comfort zone in your favourite activities?

Planning your next event:

1. What type of event are you planning, and what is the event's goal?

2. Who is your target audience, and what are their interests and preferences?

3. What logistical details must you consider, such as location, time, and budget?

4. How can you promote your event and attract attendees?

5. What are some ways to evaluate the success of your event and gather feedback for future planning?

Romance With ADHD

Managing a romantic relationship can be challenging for anyone but particularly difficult for women with ADHD. They need to communicate openly with their partner about their needs and limitations and to be upfront about their diagnosis. They may find it helpful to develop coping strategies for common ADHD symptoms, such as forgetfulness and impulsivity.

It is also important to prioritize self-care, such as getting enough sleep, exercise, and time for relaxation, as these can help to manage symptoms of ADHD and reduce stress in the relationship.

Women with ADHD may benefit from working with a therapist with experience treating this disorder, either alone or with their partner. It is important to remember that no relationship is perfect, and it is okay to ask for help and support when needed.

Here are some tips that might help manage your relationship better:

- **Understand your ADHD.** Educate yourself on how ADHD affects you and how it may impact your relationships. Be honest with yourself about your struggles, but also recognize your strengths.

- **Communicate with your partner.** Let your partner know about your diagnosis and how it affects you. Be open and honest about your struggles and what you need from them. Work together to find solutions to any challenges that may arise.
- **Set goals and routines.** Develop a routine that includes time for your relationship. Set goals together and prioritize the important things for both of you. This will help you stay organized and focused.

- **Use reminders and timers.** Use alarms, reminders, and timers to help you stay on track with appointments, dates, and other commitments. This will help you avoid forgetting important things and reduce stress and anxiety.

- **Practice mindfulness.** Mindfulness practices, such as deep breathing and meditation, can help you stay focused and calm. This can be particularly helpful when you are feeling overwhelmed or stressed.

- **Seek professional support.** Consider seeing a therapist or counsellor who has experience working with ADHD. They can provide support and guidance and help you develop coping strategies.

Managing ADHD in a romantic relationship is an ongoing process. Every relationship is unique; what works for one couple may not work for another. Be patient with yourself and your partner, and keep trying different strategies until you find what works for you. You can create a happy and healthy relationship by using these strategies and working together.

◆ ◆ ◆

Key Takeaways

- ADHD can impact your ability to communicate, listen, and remember important details, making it challenging to maintain healthy relationships.
- Recognize where you excel and struggle in relationships, and work to improve in areas that may cause tension or conflict.
- Be clear and concise when expressing your feelings and thoughts, and actively listen to others to ensure you understand their perspective.
- Learn to manage your ADHD symptoms in healthy ways, such as through exercise, meditation, and therapy, to reduce stress and improve your relationships.
- Accept feedback from loved ones and be willing to change how you approach relationships to strengthen them.

Suppose you want to learn more about managing your physical health with ADHD. In that case, I encourage you to continue reading the next chapter. You will find a wealth of information and tips for improving your physical well-being, managing your symptoms, and living your best life with ADHD.

◆ ◆ ◆

CHAPTER 7: MY PHYSICAL HEALTH AND ADHD

Managing ADHD requires a holistic approach that includes physical health, such as regular exercise, adequate sleep, and balanced nutrition. –Dr. Sharon Saline.

When we think of ADHD, we often think of its impact on our mental health and daily functioning. However, did you know that ADHD can also significantly impact your physical health? From poor sleep and nutrition to high-stress levels and a sedentary lifestyle, ADHD can make it challenging to maintain a healthy body.

In this chapter, we will explore the connection

between ADHD, your physical health, and practical strategies for improving your wellness.

You will learn how to develop healthy habits that support your mind and body, from sleep hygiene and exercise to nutrition and stress reduction. By the end of this chapter, you will be well-equipped to take charge of your physical health and feel your best every day.

While ADHD is often associated with hyperactivity, inattention, and impulsivity, it can also impact other areas of a person's life, including their eating habits. Research suggests that women with ADHD are more prone to developing disordered eating habits like binge eating, emotional eating, and other unhealthy patterns(Rucklidge & Johnston, 2020).

One possible explanation for this is the effect of ADHD on executive functioning skills. These skills are responsible for planning, organizing, and regulating behaviours related to food and eating.

Women with ADHD may have difficulty with impulsivity, emotional dysregulation, and poor self-control around food, which can lead to disordered eating habits. For example, they may find it challenging to resist impulsive food choices, need help stopping eating when full, or find it challenging to plan and prepare healthy meals.

Moreover, some women with ADHD may use food to self-medicate or cope with negative emotions. Stress, anxiety, and depression occur daily among women with ADHD, and these emotions can lead to overeating or choosing unhealthy food to feel better in the short term. Emotional eating, which involves eating to soothe or cope with emotions, can be particularly problematic for women with ADHD.

The intersection of ADHD and eating habits can significantly impact a woman's overall health and well-being. Women with ADHD may be at an increased risk of developing health problems such as obesity, diabetes, and heart disease due to their eating habits. In addition, disordered eating habits can exacerbate ADHD symptoms and decrease quality of life.

However, it is essential to note that not all women with ADHD will struggle with disordered eating habits. Many women with ADHD can maintain healthy eating habits through self-awareness, planning, and seeking support from healthcare professionals or loved ones. Developing strategies such as meal planning, setting regular mealtimes, and practicing mindful eating can help manage disordered eating habits.

If you are struggling with an eating habit disorder, seeking the support of a healthcare professional can be helpful. A therapist or registered dietitian can guide developing healthy eating habits while managing your symptoms. Creating a support system that includes loved ones who can provide emotional support and encouragement is essential.

Eating Habits and ADHD

While there is no specific diet for ADHD, eating a well-balanced, nutrient-rich diet may help manage symptoms. Here are some examples of healthy foods that may be beneficial for women with ADHD:

1. Fatty fish (salmon, tuna, mackerel) are rich in Omega-3 fatty acids that support brain function.
2. Whole grains (brown rice, quinoa, and whole wheat bread) provide a slow release of energy, which can help maintain focus and concentration.
3. Lean protein (chicken, turkey, lean beef, and eggs) provides amino acids essential for neurotransmitter function.
4. Fruits and vegetables (berries, apples, broccoli, and spinach) provide essential vitamins and antioxidants for brain health.

5. Nuts and seeds (almonds, walnuts, and pumpkin seeds) provide healthy fats and nutrients that support brain function.
6. Legumes (beans, lentils, and chickpeas) provide protein, fibre, and complex carbohydrates that support steady energy levels and brain function.
7. Low-fat dairy (milk, yogurt, and cheese) provides calcium and protein essential for overall health and brain function.

It is important to note that each woman with ADHD may have different dietary needs and sensitivities, so it is always best to consult a healthcare professional or registered dietitian to create a personalized plan.

A balanced diet is essential for overall health and can support ADHD symptoms. However, limited evidence supports specific vitamins or supplements for treating ADHD. However, here are some vitamins that are important for overall brain health and may be beneficial for women with ADHD:

1. **Omega-3 Fatty Acids:** These healthy fats can be found in fatty fish, flaxseeds, chia seeds, and walnuts. Omega-3s play an essential role in brain function and development. They may help improve attention and reduce hyperactivity in

children with ADHD.

2. **Iron:** Iron is an essential nutrient for brain development and function. Good sources of iron include red meat, seafood, beans, lentils, poultry, and leafy green vegetables. Iron deficiency can cause fatigue, irritability, and difficulty concentrating.
3. **Zinc:** Zinc is an essential mineral for neurotransmitter function and can help support cognitive function. Good sources of zinc include oysters, chicken, beef, pork, beans, nuts, and whole grains.
4. **Vitamin D:** Vitamin D is essential for bones and may affect cognitive function. Sunlight is the best source of vitamin D, but it can also be found in fortified foods such as milk, orange juice, and cereal.

Although these vitamins may benefit overall brain health, they must not be used as a substitute for prescribed medication or therapy for ADHD. Always consult a healthcare professional or registered dietitian before starting a new supplement regimen.

Benefits of Workout

As we have discussed, women with ADHD often have difficulty with attention, hyperactivity, and impulsivity, which impacts their academic, occupational, and social functioning. While medication and therapy are commonly used to manage symptoms of ADHD, research has shown that exercise can also play a critical role in improving outcomes (Berwid & Halperin, 2012).

One of the primary benefits of exercise for women with ADHD is its impact on executive function. Research has consistently shown that women with ADHD have impairments in executive function, and these deficits can significantly impact their ability to function in daily life. However, exercise has improved executive function in women with ADHD. In a study published in the Journal of Attention Disorders (2018), researchers found that 20 minutes of moderate-intensity exercise significantly improved working memory, inhibition, and cognitive flexibility in women with ADHD.

Another benefit of exercise for women with ADHD is its impact on mood and behaviour. Women with ADHD are at increased risk for developing mood disorders, such as anxiety and depression, which can further impair their ability to function.

However, exercise has been shown to improve mood and reduce symptoms of anxiety and depression. Researchers have found that exercise programs significantly improve mood and reduce anxiety and depression symptoms in women with

ADHD (Di Trani et al., 2018).

Exercise can provide a way to regulate hyperactivity and impulsivity. Many women with ADHD struggle with restlessness and impulsivity, leading to difficulties in social situations and academic or occupational settings. However, exercise provides an outlet for this energy, allowing women with ADHD to channel their hyperactivity constructively and beneficially. Also, exercise has been shown to improve attention and focus, which can help them better regulate their behaviour and make more thoughtful decisions.

ADHD and Sports

Exercise is an essential component of a holistic approach to managing ADHD symptoms. The benefits of exercise for women with ADHD include improvements in executive function, mood, and behaviour regulation. Incorporating regular exercise into the daily routine can significantly improve their quality of life and overall functioning. Some examples of exercises and sports that may be well-suited for women with ADHD:

- **Dancing**: Dancing is a fun and high-energy way to get moving and burn calories. Plus, it is a great way to improve coordination, balance, and rhythm. Try a dance class, turn up your favourite music, and dance around your living room.

- *Yoga* is a low-impact exercise that can help reduce stress, increase flexibility, and improve focus. Some forms of yoga, such as Vinyasa, can also be quite physically demanding, providing a good workout for the body.
- **Martial arts:** Many women with ADHD enjoy martial arts because they provide a structured and disciplined environment. Martial arts also offer a great way to improve coordination, balance, and self-defence skills. Consider trying out a class in karate, jiu-jitsu, or taekwondo.
- **Hiking**: Going out into nature and hiking can significantly improve focus and reduce stress. Hiking also provides an excellent cardiovascular workout and can be done alone or with friends.
- **Swimming**: Swimming is a low-impact exercise that can provide an excellent workout for the entire body. It is a great way to reduce anxiety and stress. Consider joining a local swim team or hitting your local pool for a solo swim.
- **Rock climbing:** Rock climbing can provide a great physical and mental challenge for women with ADHD. It requires focus, strength, and problem-solving skills. Consider trying a local rock climbing gym or signing up for an outdoor climbing adventure.

- **Team sports:** For some women with ADHD, team sports can significantly improve social skills and build self-confidence. Consider joining a local soccer, basketball, or volleyball team.
- **Pilates**: Pilates is a low-impact exercise that builds core strength, improves flexibility, and enhances balance. It can be done alone or in a group class.
- **Running**: Running is a great way to improve cardiovascular health and burn calories. For women with ADHD, it can also be an excellent way to improve focus and reduce stress. Consider joining a local running club or simply hitting the pavement alone.

The best exercise for you is one you enjoy and can stick with over the long term. Experiment with different activities and find what works best for you!

◆ ◆ ◆

Key Takeaways

- Regular exercise and physical activity can benefit women with ADHD, including improved mood, reduced stress and anxiety, and better sleep.
- Developing healthy eating habits and a balanced diet can help manage symptoms of ADHD and improve overall health and well-being.
- Strategies for improving time management and organization can help women with ADHD prioritize self-care activities, such as exercise and meal planning, into their daily routines.
- While living with ADHD can be challenging, developing healthy habits and strategies for physical well-being can help improve quality of life and overall functioning.

If you wish to learn more about how ADHD can impact your career as a woman, I recommend reading the next chapter, "Women With ADHD and Careers." In this chapter, you will gain insights into the unique challenges that women with ADHD face in the workplace, and you will learn strategies to help you thrive professionally despite your condition.

The chapter covers identifying your strengths and weaknesses, setting realistic goals, managing time, prioritizing tasks, developing coping strategies, and seeking accommodations and support when necessary. By the end of the chapter, you will better understand how to maximize your potential and achieve success in your career as a woman with ADHD.

◆ ◆ ◆

CHAPTER 8: ADHD AND CAREERS

Being a successful woman with ADHD means embracing and using your quirks to your advantage. –Sari Solden

ADHD can present unique challenges when managing your career, from difficulties with organization and time management to distractibility and restlessness in the workplace. However, with the right strategies and mindset, ADHD can offer unique advantages to help you excel in your career.

This chapter will explore how to navigate the workplace with ADHD, from finding the right job and managing your workload to communicating with your boss and colleagues.

You will learn how to leverage your ADHD strengths to thrive in your career and overcome the common obstacles that can arise. By the end of this chapter, you will have the tools you need to take your career to the next level while honoring your unique ADHD wiring.

Women diagnosed with ADHD may face discrimination and stigma in the workplace, mainly if their symptoms are severe. Some women may feel ashamed or embarrassed about their ADHD diagnosis, affecting their self-confidence and ability to speak up in the workplace. Women with this condition may feel that they have to work harder than their peers to achieve the same level of success, and they may struggle to gain recognition for their accomplishments.

On the other hand, some women may have ADHD without realizing it. Many women with ADHD go undiagnosed, particularly if they have primarily inattentive symptoms rather than hyperactive or impulsive ones.

Women with undiagnosed ADHD may struggle to keep up with the demands of their job, and they may feel overwhelmed or anxious. They may have trouble staying organized, managing their time, or completing tasks on time, making them feel like they are not meeting their potential. They might also have difficulty with interpersonal relationships in the workplace, as they might be seen as disorganized or forgetful.

For women who are aware of their ADHD diagnosis, several strategies can help them succeed in the workplace. One of the most important strategies is to seek support from colleagues, supervisors, or a therapist. Women with ADHD may benefit from having a mentor or coach who can provide guidance and feedback on their work.

They may also benefit from accommodations such as flexible work hours, extra time to complete tasks, or the ability to work from home. They can also benefit from strategies such as breaking tasks into smaller pieces, using a planner or calendar to stay organized, and taking frequent breaks to avoid burnout.

Working in a Survival Job

ADHD can make working a survival job, paying bills, and managing day-to-day responsibilities challenging. However, with the right mindset and strategies, it is possible to make this a short-term situation and have a bigger plan for the future.

It is essential to understand that having ADHD can

make it harder to focus, prioritize, and manage time. This can make it challenging to perform well in a survival job, such as working in retail or food service. However, it is crucial to remember that a survival job is temporary and a means to an end.

To make it a short-term situation, it is essential to have a plan in place. This plan should include steps toward a career that aligns with your passions and strengths. This could include returning to school, taking online courses, or working with a career coach.

It is also essential to have a support system in place. This can include family, friends, or a therapist who can help you stay focused, motivated, and on track toward your goals. It is essential to have people who can help you stay accountable and celebrate your successes.

Additionally, it is essential to create a routine that works for you. This could include setting a daily schedule, breaking tasks into smaller chunks, and using tools like timers and reminders to stay on track. It is also helpful to prioritize tasks and tackle the most critical ones. One way to make a survival job more manageable is to find ways to incorporate your strengths and interests into your work. This could include taking on additional responsibilities that align with your passions or finding ways to make your tasks more engaging and challenging.

Taking care of your physical and mental health is also essential. Exercise, sleep, and proper nutrition can help you stay focused, energized, and motivated. Take more breaks and practice self-care to avoid burnout. It is essential to have a plan, support system, and routine that works for you and a focus on your strengths and passions. With these tools, you can overcome the challenges of ADHD and create a fulfilling career and life for yourself.

Set Long-Term Career Goals

Setting long-term career goals is essential for achieving your desired professional success. Here are some techniques to guide you in setting your long-term career goals:

- **Identify your interests**: Start by identifying the areas of work that interest you the most. This will help you focus on a career path that aligns with your passions and talents.
- **Set achievable goals:** It is essential to set measurable, achievable, and challenging goals. Break down your long-term career goals into smaller, more manageable milestones, and set specific deadlines for achieving them.
- **Research career paths:** Research the career paths that interest you. This will help you determine what skills and qualifications

you need to achieve your long-term career goals. Look for job descriptions, educational and experience requirements, and career advancement opportunities.

- **Develop a plan:** Once you have identified your long-term career goals, develop a plan. This plan should include the steps you need to take, the resources you need to acquire, and the timeline for completing each step.
- **Stay flexible:** Your long-term career goals may change as you gain new experiences and develop new interests. Be flexible and open to change, and modify your goals as necessary.
- **Network:** Building a professional network is essential for achieving long-term career goals. Attend industry events, connect with people on LinkedIn, and build relationships with mentors and colleagues who can help you advance your career.
- **Measure progress:** Regularly assess your progress toward your long-term career goals, celebrate your achievements, and use setbacks as opportunities to learn and grow.

By following these techniques, you can set long-term career goals that are achievable, realistic, and aligned with your passions and interests. Setting long-term career goals is an ongoing process that requires dedication, hard work, and adaptability.

Embracing ADHD at Work

For women with ADHD, managing their symptoms at work can be challenging. However, with the right strategies, women with ADHD can use their unique strengths to excel in the workplace.
One way women with ADHD can use their condition positively is by embracing their creativity. Many women with this disorder have a natural ability to think outside the box and find other innovative solutions to problems. Their creativity can be valuable in any workplace, whether in the arts, sciences, or business.

Another way to use ADHD positively at work is to embrace hyperfocus. Although ADHD is often associated with distractibility, some people can also experience periods of intense focus on a particular task or project. Women with ADHD can use this hyperfocus to their advantage by scheduling their work to allow them to focus on their most important tasks during these periods of heightened concentration.

Women can also leverage their ability to multitask to their advantage. While multitasking is not always an efficient way to work, it can be an effective strategy. Working on multiple tasks simultaneously, women with ADHD can prevent boredom and stay engaged, increasing productivity and job satisfaction.

Also, there are benefits to developing a routine and structure. Establishing a routine can help them stay organized and focused and minimize the potential for distraction. Additionally, breaking down larger projects into smaller, more manageable tasks can help women with ADHD prioritize their work and prevent becoming overwhelmed.

Women with ADHD can benefit from seeking out accommodations in the workplace. Under the Americans with Disabilities Act (ADA), employers must provide reasonable accommodations to individuals with disabilities, including ADHD. Accommodations can include flexible work hours, noise-cancelling headphones, or written instructions in addition to verbal instructions.

Tips to Improve Relationship With Your Career

ADHD can present multiple challenges for women in the workplace. However, many strategies and tips can help women with ADHD improve their relationships with their careers. Here are a few suggestions:

- **Identify your strengths and weaknesses:** It is essential to identify your strengths, weaknesses, and any triggers that might make it difficult to focus or stay organized. This can help you find a job or career path that plays to your strengths and minimizes your weaknesses.

- **Create a routine:** Daily routines can help you stay on track and avoid feeling overwhelmed. Make sure to include regular breaks and set specific times for tasks you must complete.
- **Use tools and technology:** Many tools and technologies are available to help with organization, time management, and productivity. Consider using a planner or task management app to keep track of your schedule and deadlines.
- **Advocate for yourself:** Be bold and speak up and advocate for the support you need in the workplace, such as accommodations or additional resources. This can include a quiet workspace or extra time to complete tasks.
- **Find a supportive environment:** Seek out a work environment that understands and supports your needs. Look for employers or colleagues willing to help you create a work environment conducive to your success.
- **Get organized:** Use colour coding, labelling, and decluttering tools to organize your workspace and projects. This can help you stay focused and avoid distractions.
- **Use your creativity:** Many women with ADHD are creative and have unique ideas. Use this to your advantage in your career and find ways to channel your creativity into your

work.

ADHD can be a strength as well as a challenge. By identifying your strengths, creating a routine, using tools and technology, advocating for yourself, finding a supportive environment, getting organized, and using your creativity, you can succeed in your career despite the challenges of ADHD.

◆ ◆ ◆

Date ---------

Exercise 24

Here are some questions you could ask yourself to find the right career for you:

1. What are your strengths and weaknesses?

2. What are your interests and passions?

3. What are your core values?

4. What kind of work environment do you thrive in?

5. What type of work schedule do you prefer?

6. What kind of tasks or activities do you find engaging and motivating?

7. What kind of tasks or activities do you find challenging or overwhelming?

8. Are you more of a big-picture thinker or detail-oriented?

9. Do you prefer working independently or in a team?

10. What support and accommodations do you need to perform at your best?

These questions can help a woman with ADHD identify her strengths, weaknesses, preferences, and career needs. Moreover, it can be helpful to consult with a career counsellor or coach who has experience working with individuals with ADHD to get personalized guidance and support.

Best Jobs for ADHD Minds

Women with ADHD have unique strengths and

challenges that may make some jobs more suitable. Here are some potential job options for women with ADHD:

- **Entrepreneur**: Starting a business can provide the flexibility and autonomy many people with ADHD need to succeed. As an entrepreneur, you can choose a field that aligns with your interests and strengths and set your schedule and work style.
- **Creative fields:** Jobs such as writing, graphic design, or photography can be well-suited to people with ADHD. These jobs often require high creativity and can offer much variety and stimulation.
- **Healthcare:** Jobs in healthcare, such as nursing or occupational therapy, can be a good fit for women with ADHD. These jobs require a high level of attention to detail and often involve much problem-solving, which can be stimulating for people with this disorder.
- **Education:** Teaching or working in education can also be a good option for women with ADHD. These jobs often require a lot of energy and creativity and can offer variety and stimulation.
- **Sales or marketing:** Jobs in sales or marketing can be well-suited to people with ADHD, as they often involve much social interaction and require a high level of energy and creativity.

This is a tiny sampling of the many job options available to women with ADHD. Choosing a job that aligns with your interests and strengths is as important as finding a work environment that supports your needs. It is also essential to communicate with your employer about any accommodations you may need to be successful in your job.

How to Stay Motivated at Work

Staying motivated at work while having ADHD can be a challenge, but several strategies can help. Breaking tasks into smaller steps, setting goals and priorities, using reminders and alarms, taking regular breaks, minimizing distractions, using visual aids, and celebrating achievements can help maintain focus and motivation. It is essential to find what works best for you and to experiment with different strategies. Seeking support from a doctor or therapist may provide additional resources and strategies to manage ADHD symptoms and stay motivated at work.

◆ ◆ ◆

Date ---------

Exercise 25

Here are some tips that may help you stay motivated and focused:

- **Break tasks into smaller steps:** This will help you feel less overwhelmed, work more manageably, and make starting easier.
- **Set goals and prioritize:** Setting clear goals for what you want to accomplish each day and prioritizing your tasks will help you focus on the most important things first.
- **Use reminders and alarms:** Using reminders and alarms to help you stay on track will help you remember important meetings, deadlines, and tasks.
- **Take breaks:** Regular breaks will help you stay refreshed and avoid burnout. This will help you maintain your focus and energy throughout the day.
- **Minimize distractions:** Turn off notifications and alerts on your phone and computer. You may also find noise-cancelling headphones or working in a quiet space beneficial.
- **Use visual aids:** Calendars, to-do lists, and mind maps can help you stay organized and

focused.

- **Reward yourself:** Celebrate your achievements, no matter how small. Recognizing your accomplishments can help you stay motivated and positive.

Every woman with ADHD is unique, and what works for one may not work for another. Experimenting with different strategies and finding what works best for you is essential. Consider talking to your doctor or therapist about additional strategies and resources that may help you manage your ADHD symptoms at work.

◆ ◆ ◆

Key Takeaways

- Choosing a career that aligns with one's strengths and interests can increase motivation and job satisfaction for women with ADHD.
- Open communication with employers and colleagues about one's diagnosis can help to dispel misconceptions and build understanding and support.
- Developing routines, schedules, and organizational systems can help women with ADHD manage their workload and meet deadlines.
- Seeking accommodations, such as flexible work hours or a quiet workspace, can help women with ADHD perform their best.

The next chapter, "My Finance and ADHD," provides practical tips and tools to help you handle your money, including how to set financial goals, create a budget, manage debt, and save for the future. By following the advice in this chapter, you can take control of your finances and feel more confident about your financial future. So, take the next step and read on to learn how to manage your money with ADHD!

◆ ◆ ◆

CHAPTER 9: MY FINANCE AND ADHD

Money talks, but for those with ADHD, it can be hard to listen. Effective money management requires more than just numbers; it takes discipline, focus, and a strategic approach to overcome the distractions and impulsivity of ADHD. –Anonymous

Managing personal finances can be a challenge for anyone, but for those with ADHD, it can feel incredibly daunting. From impulsive spending and disorganization to difficulty tracking expenses and sticking to a budget, this disorder can make it challenging to achieve financial stability. However, taking control of your finances and achieving your goals is possible with the right strategies and tools.

This chapter will explore practical strategies for managing your finances with ADHD, from creating a budget and tracking your expenses to reducing impulse spending and developing healthy financial habits. By the end of this chapter, you will be well-equipped to take charge of your finances and achieve financial success.
The impulsive behaviour and lack of organization often come with ADHD can lead to overspending, missed payments, and other financial problems. However, developing good financial planning skills can bring significant benefits to women with ADHD. Effective financial planning can help these women manage their money, reduce stress, and achieve their financial goals.

One of the primary benefits of financial planning is improved financial stability. This can be achieved through setting a budget, tracking expenses, and creating a plan for debt reduction.

When financial planning skills are developed and practiced, it can help women with ADHD manage their money more effectively and maintain their financial stability. By managing their finances more effectively, they can avoid unnecessary debt, build wealth, and achieve their financial goals.

Another benefit of financial planning is stress reduction. Financial struggles can be a significant source of stress, and poor financial management can worsen this problem. However, by creating a financial plan, women with ADHD can reduce stress and gain peace of mind by knowing their finances are in order.

They can set a budget, prioritize bills, and plan for upcoming expenses to avoid last-minute surprises that can be stressful for anyone but particularly challenging for women with an ADHD diagnosis.

Effective financial planning can help develop better time-management habits. By prioritizing financial tasks and managing money effectively, they can overcome procrastination and improve their time management skills. When they learn to prioritize their financial duties, they can focus on the most important tasks and cut unnecessary expenses. This can help them develop better time-management habits and reduce their stress levels.

Financial planning can help women with ADHD achieve their financial goals. When they develop a budget and plan for debt reduction, they can begin to work toward their financial goals, such as saving for a down payment on a home or paying off credit card debt. By working toward their goals, they can build confidence and self-esteem, which can help them in other areas of their lives.

How Do I Deal With My Money?

For women with ADHD, setting and achieving financial goals can be a challenging task. It is essential to establish realistic financial goals that are specific, measurable, achievable, relevant, and time-bound (SMART goals). The best way to achieve financial goals is to create a budget that reflects your income and expenses. They can consider using visual aids, such as charts or graphs, to help them better understand their finances.

Another critical step is to automate payments and savings to avoid missed payments or impulse purchases. They can also seek professional help from a financial advisor or therapist specializing in this disorder to create a customized financial plan that meets their unique needs and challenges.

With patience, determination, and the proper support, women with ADHD can successfully achieve their financial goals and secure their futures. However, there are some strategies you can use to help manage your finances effectively. Here are a few tips:

- **Set up automatic payments:** One way to avoid missed payments is to set up automatic payments for bills and other expenses. This can help ensure that bills are paid on time, even if you forget or get distracted.

- **Use reminders and alerts:** If you cannot set up automatic payments, use reminders and alerts to help you remember to pay bills on time. You can set reminders on your phone or computer or use a budgeting app that sends notifications when bills are due.
- **Simplify your finances:** It is helpful to simplify your finances as much as possible. This might mean consolidating bank accounts, reducing the number of credit cards you have, or using a budgeting app to track all your expenses in one place.
- **Set a budget:** A budget can help you stay on track and avoid overspending. When creating a budget, include all your expenses, including bills, groceries, and other regular costs.
- **Get professional help:** If you are having trouble managing your finances, consider getting professional help from a financial planner or therapist specializing in ADHD. They can help you create a personalized plan to manage your finances and provide guidance and support.

Overall, managing finances can be a challenge for anyone, but women with ADHD may face additional hurdles. By taking a proactive approach and implementing some of these strategies, you can take control of your finances and improve your financial well-being.

Be On Top of All Expenses

Monitoring your spending and staying on top of your expenses can help you make better financial decisions and achieve your goals. First, you should create a budget to identify your income and expenses. This will help determine how much money you can allocate to different categories such as rent, groceries, entertainment, and savings. Once you have a budget, you can use different tools to track your spending, such as a spreadsheet or a budgeting app. You should also keep all your receipts and record all your transactions.

Setting short and long-term goals can help you achieve financial stability and reach your objectives over time. Review your spending regularly to see where you might be overspending or where you can make adjustments to stay within your budget. Always be disciplined and stick to your budget to ensure you are on top of all expenses and on track toward achieving your financial goals.

◆ ◆ ◆

Date ---------

Exercise 26

Some steps to help you set short-term and long-term financial goals:

Short-Term Financial Goals:

1. **Determine your current financial situation:** Before setting any financial goals, it is essential to understand your current financial situation. This includes understanding your income, expenses, debts, and assets.
2. **Identify your priorities:** Identify the areas where you need to focus your attention in the short term. It could be reducing your debt, increasing your savings, or managing your expenses.
3. **Set achievable and measurable goals:** Ensure that your short-term financial goals are specific, measurable, achievable, relevant, and time-bound (SMART). For example, you might set a goal to pay off a credit card debt of $2,000 in three months by paying $667 each month.
4. **Monitor your progress:** Monitor your

progress regularly and adjust your plan accordingly. Keep track of your spending and saving to ensure that you are on track to meet your short-term financial goals.

Long-Term Financial Goals:

1. **Determine your financial vision:** Start by thinking about what you want your financial future to look like. Identify your long-term objectives and the lifestyle you want to have in the future.
2. **Break down your goals:** Once you have identified your financial vision, break it into smaller, achievable milestones. For example, if the goal is to save $500,000 for retirement, break it down into smaller, achievable milestones like saving $50,000 in five years.
3. **Set achievable and measurable goals:** Like short-term goals, ensure that your long-term financial goals are specific, measurable, achievable, relevant, and time-bound (SMART). For example, if the goal is to save $50,000 in five years, you would need to save $10,000 per year or $833 per month.
4. **Review and adjust your plan:** Regularly review your long-term financial goals and adjust if and when necessary. Factors like changes in income, expenses, or

investments may require you to adjust your goals and timeline.

Setting short- and long-term financial goals requires a clear understanding of your current financial situation, priorities, and vision for the future. Once you have established your goals, monitoring your progress regularly and adjusting your plan to ensure that you achieve financial success over time is essential.

How to Deal With Debt Effectively

Dealing with debt can lead to anxiety, depression, and constant worry about money, negatively impacting mental health. Debt can also have a long-term financial impact, as high-interest rates can result in paying significantly more over time than the original debt. Balancing debt repayment with other financial priorities, such as retirement savings or emergencies, can be challenging. Dealing with debt can be difficult and stressful. However, there are several tips you can use to help reduce your debt and regain financial control.

◆ ◆ ◆

Date ---------

Exercise 27

Here are some steps to consider:

1. **Create a budget:** The first step in reducing debt is to create a budget. List your income sources and expenses to identify where your money is going. From there, you can identify areas where you can cut back on costs and redirect that money toward debt repayment.
2. **Prioritize debt repayment:** Determine which debts have the highest interest rates and prioritize those for repayment first. By paying off the highest interest rate debt, you can reduce the interest you will pay over time.
3. **Consider debt consolidation:** If you have multiple debts with high-interest rates, consider consolidating them into a single loan with a lower interest rate. This can reduce your monthly payments and make it easier to manage your debt.
4. **Negotiate with creditors:** If you are having trouble making payments, contact your creditors and explain your situation.

They may be willing to work with you on a payment plan or offer a settlement to reduce your debt.

5. **Cut back on expenses:** To free up more money for debt repayment, look for areas where you can cut back on expenses. This might mean reducing dining out, cancelling subscriptions or memberships, or shopping for cheaper alternatives.
6. **Consider additional income:** If you struggle to make ends meet, consider working part-time or freelancing to earn additional income. This extra money can go directly toward debt repayment.
7. **Stay disciplined:** Reducing debt takes time and effort, so staying disciplined and committed to your plan is essential. Stick to your budget and make regular debt payments to achieve your financial goals.

If not managed correctly, dealing with debt can lead to a cycle of borrowing, further increasing the amount owed. While addressing debt is essential, it is crucial to consider seeking help, if necessary, to navigate the process successfully.

How to Deal With Plastics (Credit Cards)

Credit cards can be a valuable tool for managing your finances. However, it is essential to use them responsibly to avoid accumulating debt you cannot afford to pay off.

◆ ◆ ◆

Date ---------

Exercise 28

Here are some tips for dealing with credit cards effectively:

1. **Set a budget:** Make a budget for your monthly expenses and stick to it. This will help you avoid overspending and accumulating debt that you cannot afford to repay.
2. **Pay your balance in full:** Pay your credit card balance monthly to avoid costly interest charges. If you cannot pay off the balance, pay more than the minimum payment to reduce the interest charges.
3. **Keep an eye on your credit limit:** Be aware of your credit limit and avoid maxing out your card. Using too much of your available credit can negatively impact your credit score.
4. **Review your statements:** Regularly review your credit card statements to identify errors or fraudulent transactions. If you notice any unauthorized charges, report them to your card issuer immediately.

5. **Only apply for a few credit cards:** Avoid applying for too many, which can hurt your credit score. Only apply for credit cards that you need and that you can manage responsibly.

Long-Term Financial Goals

Determining long-term financial goals for women with ADHD can be challenging but essential for their financial well-being. Attention Deficit/ Hyperactivity Disorder can make it difficult to focus on long-term planning, and impulsivity can lead to excessive spending or investing.

Below are some guidelines women with ADHD can follow to develop a clear financial plan, stay focused on their long-term goals, and achieve more excellent financial stability:

- **Start with a vision:** Begin by thinking about your long-term financial aspirations. This could include buying a house, saving for retirement, paying off debt, or starting a business. A clear vision of your long-term financial goals can help you stay motivated and focused.
- **Break down goals into manageable steps:** Once you have a vision, break it down into smaller, achievable steps. For example, if you want to save $10,000 for a down payment on a house, break it down into smaller,

weekly, or monthly savings goals. This can make the process less overwhelming and more manageable.

- **Focus on one goal at a time:** Trying to achieve too many goals simultaneously can be overwhelming, especially for women with ADHD. Focus on one goal at a time, and once you have completed it, move on to the next one.
- **Work with a financial planner:** A financial planner can help you build a plan and stay accountable. They can also guide investment options, debt management, and retirement planning.
- **Regularly review and adjust goals:** ADHD symptoms can fluctuate, so reviewing and adjusting your goals as many times as needed is essential. This can help ensure your financial plan aligns with your current needs and circumstances.
- **Celebrate your achievements:** Celebrate when you achieve your financial goals, no matter how small. This can help keep you motivated and engaged in the process.

Take Control of Your Money

Tracking your spending and developing a monthly budget can be a great way to take control of your finances and ensure you are progressing toward your financial goals.

◆ ◆ ◆

Date ---------

Exercise 29

Here are the steps you can follow:

1. **Start by tracking your spending:** Keep track of your money for at least a month. You will want to track your expenses, including bills, groceries, transportation, entertainment, and any other costs you have. This can be done manually or through an app.
2. **Categorize your spending:** Once you have a record of your expenses, start categorizing them. For example, you might have housing, transportation, food, entertainment, and savings categories.
3. **Calculate your monthly income:** Determine how much money you earn each month after taxes.
4. **Set financial goals:** Decide what you want to achieve with your money. You can pay off debt, save for a vacation, or build an emergency fund.
5. **Create a budget:** Use the information you gathered in steps 1-4 to create a budget. Start by allocating your income to your

different expense categories. Be sure to prioritize your financial goals.

6. **Adjust your budget as necessary:** Your budget should be flexible and adapt to your income and expenses changes. To stay on track, make adjustments as needed.
7. **Monitor your spending:** Track it monthly and compare it to your budget. This will help you stay on track and make any necessary adjustments.
8. **Review and refine your budget:** Review your budget and make any necessary changes at the end of each month. Over time, you will become more familiar with your spending habits and be able to create a more accurate budget.

Key Takeaways

- Developing a budget and financial plan can help women with ADHD take control of their finances and avoid overspending.
- Automating bills and payments, such as setting up auto-pay for monthly bills, can help women with this disorder avoid missed payments and late fees.
- Limiting access to credit cards and other forms of credit can help women with ADHD avoid impulsive spending and accumulating debt.
- Tracking spending, either manually or with budgeting software or apps, can help them stay mindful of their spending habits and make necessary adjustments.

If you want to learn more about effective treatments for ADHD, the next chapter, "How Can I Treat ADHD?" is the perfect place to start. From medication and therapy to lifestyle changes and alternative treatments, this chapter covers everything you need to know to take control of your ADHD and thrive. You will discover a range of proven strategies and therapies that can help you manage your symptoms and live a more fulfilling life. Do not miss this valuable information–read the next chapter now!

◆◆◆

CHAPTER 10: HOW CAN I TREAT ADHD?

ADHD is not a curse or a blessing but a difference that can be directed toward whichever goals we set for ourselves. –Dr. Edward Hallowell

If you are living with ADHD, you know it can impact every aspect of your life, from your daily routines to your relationships and career. However, the good news is that a variety of effective treatments can help you manage your symptoms and improve the quality of your life.

This chapter will explore the various treatment options for ADHD, from medication and therapy to lifestyle changes and alternative approaches.

We will discuss each option's benefits and potential drawbacks and help you determine the best course of treatment for your unique needs. By the end of this chapter, you will have a comprehensive understanding of the various treatments available for ADHD and feel empowered to take action toward managing your symptoms and improving your quality of life.

Cognitive Behavioral Therapy (CBT)

Cognitive Behavioral Therapy is a psychotherapy that focuses on the relationships between thoughts, feelings, and behaviours. It is based on the idea that negative thoughts and behaviours can contribute to emotional problems like anxiety and depression.

The therapy is designed to help individuals identify negative thinking and behaviour patterns contributing to their problems. It involves working with a therapist to identify negative thoughts and behaviours and develop strategies to replace them with positive ones. This might include learning to recognize and challenge negative thoughts, practicing relaxation techniques, and developing new coping strategies.

CBT is a time-limited therapy that typically lasts between 12 and 20 sessions. It is a structured and goal-oriented therapy that provides the tools and skills to manage thoughts and behaviours more effectively and improve mental health and well-being. It effectively treats various mental health conditions, including anxiety disorders, depression, Post-Traumatic Stress Disorder (PTSD), and Obsessive-Compulsive Disorder (OCD).

For women with ADHD, this type of therapy can be beneficial in addressing the unique challenges they face. These challenges may include time management, organization, impulsivity, emotional regulation, and self-esteem. Through CBT, women with ADHD can learn to identify negative thoughts and behaviours and develop more effective coping strategies. For example, they may learn to break down tasks into smaller, more manageable steps, use planners and timers to stay organized, and practice relaxation techniques to manage stress and anxiety.

Research has shown that CBT can significantly improve ADHD symptoms and the overall quality of life for women with ADHD (Lopez et al., 2018). By addressing negative thought patterns and developing effective coping strategies, women with ADHD can learn to manage their symptoms better and achieve their goals.

One real-life example of the effectiveness of behavioural therapy for adults with ADHD is a study conducted by Safren and colleagues (2005). In this study, 86 adults with ADHD were randomly assigned to either a cognitive-behavioural therapy (CBT) or supportive psychotherapy (SPT) group.

The CBT group received 12 weekly therapy sessions to improve time-management skills, organization, and planning. The SPT group received 12 weekly therapy sessions focused on emotional support and validation.

The study results showed that the individuals in the CBT group significantly improved their ADHD symptoms, including reductions in distractibility, hyperactivity, and impulsivity, as well as advances in time management and organization. In addition, the individuals in the CBT group reported more excellent overall functioning and quality of life improvements than those in the SPT group.

This study proves that behavioural therapy, specifically CBT, can be a valuable treatment option for adults with ADHD. It highlights the importance of developing practical skills and strategies to help individuals manage their symptoms and improve their daily functioning.

Medications

Remember that symptoms of inattention,

hyperactivity, and impulsivity characterize ADHD. Medication, such as stimulants and non-stimulants, can be a helpful tool in managing these symptoms.

It increases the availability of neurotransmitters in the brain, such as dopamine and norepinephrine. This can improve focus, attention, and impulse control, which can help women with ADHD to be more productive and successful in their daily lives.

However, medication is not a cure for ADHD. It is important to remember that medication alone cannot eliminate all symptoms of ADHD. It is often most effective when combined with other treatments, such as therapy, lifestyle changes, and support from family and friends.

It is also important to note that medication might not be the best option for everyone with ADHD. Some medications may cause side effects. Therefore, it is recommended to take medication under the guidance of a healthcare professional, as they can help monitor its effectiveness and make adjustments as needed.

ADHD Diet and Exercise

An ADHD-friendly diet and exercise routine can help manage symptoms of the disorder. A balanced diet with plenty of whole foods, healthy fats, and lean proteins can help improve mood stability and mental focus. Regular exercise can help improve attention, reduce impulsivity, and enhance mood regulation. Exercise also promotes healthy sleep patterns and can help reduce stress and anxiety, common co-occurring conditions with ADHD.

◆ ◆ ◆

Date ---------

Exercise 30

Some tips for an ADHD-friendly diet and exercise routine:

Diet

- Avoid processed foods and sugary snacks. These can cause blood sugar levels to spike and crash, leading to mood swings and difficulty concentrating.
- Eat a balanced diet with plenty of whole grains, fruits, vegetables, and lean proteins. These foods can help stabilize blood sugar levels and promote overall health.
- Consider including more Omega-3 fatty acids in your diet. Omega-3s have been shown to have potential benefits for people with ADHD.

Exercise

- Regular exercise can help improve focus, reduce impulsivity, and regulate emotions in people with ADHD.
- Choose activities that you enjoy and that you can stick with over time. This might include

team sports, martial arts, or solo activities like running or biking.

- Aim for at least 30 minutes of exercise most days of the week. You do not need to go to the gym or do anything fancy; even a brisk walk can be beneficial.

Only diet and exercise may not be enough to manage ADHD symptoms. Still, they can be helpful with other treatments and strategies, such as medication, therapy, and organizational tools.

Healthy Eating

Healthy eating habits can be an essential part of managing symptoms of ADHD. A diet that includes nutrient-dense whole foods, healthy fats, and lean proteins can provide the body with the fuel it needs to function correctly.

A diet that is low in processed foods and high in nutrient-dense whole foods can help support brain health and reduce symptoms of ADHD. On the other hand, sugary and processed foods can cause fluctuations in blood sugar levels, leading to mood swings, difficulty concentrating, and hyperactivity. Eating regularly throughout the day is essential to maintain stable blood sugar levels and avoid skipping meals.

ADHD and Self-Care

Self-care is an essential aspect of managing symptoms of ADHD. This can include activities that help reduce stress, promote relaxation, and support overall health and well-being. Regular exercises, such as yoga, walking, or other low-impact activities, can help reduce hyperactivity and promote relaxation.

Additionally, engaging in activities that promote mindfulness, such as meditation or deep breathing exercises, can help improve focus and reduce impulsivity. Getting enough sleep is also vital for managing your symptoms.

Making time for self-care can help reduce stress, promote emotional regulation, and enhance the overall quality of life for people with ADHD. Establishing a consistent sleep schedule and creating a calming bedtime routine is essential. Other self-care practices include engaging in hobbies, connecting with supportive friends and family members, and practicing good time management skills.

◆ ◆ ◆

Key Takeaways

- There is no one-size-fits-all treatment for ADHD, and finding a treatment plan that works for you may take some trial and error.
- Some common treatments for ADHD include medication, therapy, and lifestyle changes.
- Cognitive behavioural techniques can help people with this disorder maximize rational thinking to help generate solutions.
- Lifestyle changes like exercise, a healthy diet, and good sleep habits can also help manage symptoms.
- Working with a healthcare provider to develop a treatment plan tailored to your specific needs and goals is essential.

◆ ◆ ◆

CONCLUSION

This workbook is a comprehensive guide that provides practical tools, exercises, and information to help women with ADHD thrive in all areas of their lives. It provides a step-by-step process that enables readers to create a personalized plan to help them achieve their goals and manage their symptoms effectively.

One of the key takeaways from this workbook is the importance of taking control of your life. This means not letting ADHD define you but instead developing a sense of agency over your life. Be proactive and take charge of your life by using the tools and exercises provided in the workbook to achieve your goals. You need to practice the exercises for at least seven minutes a day. The workbook emphasizes the importance of consistent practice to see tangible results. Please commit to this daily practice to make lasting changes.

The book also emphasizes the importance of seeking professional help and using the workbook.

While the exercises and tools in the workbook are helpful, they are not a substitute for professional treatment. See a therapist or other medical professional for a more comprehensive treatment plan tailored to your needs.

Thrive With Adult ADHD Workbook for Women is an invaluable resource for any woman with ADHD who wants to live her best life. By taking action and committing to daily practice of the exercises and tools provided in the workbook, you can take control of your life and manage your symptoms more effectively.

This book is a call to action for all women with ADHD to take control of their lives and thrive!

◆ ◆ ◆

REFERENCES

Berwid, O. G., & Halperin, J. M. (2012). *Emerging Support for a Role of Exercise in Attention-Deficit/Hyperactivity Disorder Intervention Planning.* Current Psychiatry Reports, 14(5), 543–551. https://doi.org/10.1007/s11920-012-0297-4

Di Trani, M., Traversa, M., Fini, V., & Schiavone, G. (2018). *Women with ADHD: A systematic review of literature.* Journal of Attention Disorders, 22(10), 877–885. https://doi.org/10.1177/1087054715607056

Hafeez, M., Kamal, A., & Malik, J. A. (2019). W*omen with ADHD: Challenges and possible solutions*. International Journal of Mental Health Systems, 13(1), 1-8. https://doi.org/10.1186/s13033-019-0273-7

Hormozi, M., Rostami, R., Rasouli, M., & Goodarzi, M. A. (2020). *The relationship between ADHD symptoms and impulsivity, depression, and anxiety in women with bipolar disorder*. Journal of Family Medicine and Primary Care, 9(5), 2402–2407. https://doi.org/10.4103/jfmpc.jfmpc_121_20

Kathleen Nadeau, K. G., & Littman, E. B. (2015).

Understanding girls with ADHD. Advantage Books.

Honos-Webb, L. (2020). *The ADHD workbook for teens: Activities to help you gain motivation and confidence*. Instant Help Books.

Lopez, P. L., Torrente, F. M., Ciapponi, A., Lischinsky, A. G., Cetkovich-Bakmas, M., Rojas, J. I., Romano, M., & Manes, F. F. (2018). *Cognitive-behavioural interventions for attention deficit hyperactivity disorder (ADHD) in adults.* Cochrane Database of Systematic Reviews, 3(3). https://doi.org/10.1002/14651858.cd010840.pub2

Matlen, T. J. (2020). *Survival tips for women with ADHD: Beyond piles, palms, and Post-its*. Specialty Press.

Mitchell, J. T., McIntyre, E. M., English, J. S., Dennis, M. F., Beckham, J. C., & Kollins, S. H. (2013). *A Pilot Trial of Mindfulness Meditation Training for ADHD in Adulthood: Impact on Core Symptoms, Executive Functioning, and Emotion Dysregulation.* Journal of Attention Disorders, 21(13), 1105–1120. https://doi.org/10.1177/1087054713513328

Mowlem, F. D., Rosenqvist, M. A., Martin, J., Lichtenstein, P., Asherson, P., & Larsson, H. (2018). *Sex differences in predicting ADHD clinical diagnosis and pharmacological treatment.* European Child & Adolescent Psychiatry, 28(4), 481–489. https://doi.org/10.1007/s00787-018-1211-3

Novotni, M. (2012). *What does everybody else know that I don't?: Social skills help for adults with attention deficit/hyperactivity disorder.* Specialty Press.

Orenstein, P. (2021). *Finding our way: Women with ADHD navigating rocky relationships, stigma, and internal struggles.* Berkley.

Quinn, P. O., & Madhoo, M. (2014). *A review of attention-deficit/hyperactivity disorder in women and girls: Uncovering this hidden diagnosis.* The Primary Care Companion for CNS Disorders, 16(3). https://doi.org/10.4088/PCC.13r01596

Quinn, P. O., Madhoo, M., Nijjar, R., & Huynh, J. (2020). *A systematic review of the experiences and perspectives of women with ADHD.* Journal of Attention Disorders, 24(11), 1487–1500. https://doi.org/10.1177/1087054720920159

Quinn, P. O. (2002). *Putting on the brakes: Young people's guide to understanding ADHD.* Magination Press.

Robin, A. L., & Souders, M. C. (2018). *ADHD and anxiety in girls.* Journal of Attention Disorders, 22(2), 178-185. https://doi.org/10.1177/1087054714547716

Rucklidge, J. J., & Johnstone, J. (2020). *Nutrient supplementation approaches in the treatment of ADHD symptoms in children and adults.* Nutrients, 12(6), 1-22. https://doi.org/10.3390/nu12061639

Sari Solden, S. (2018). *Journeys through*

ADDulthood: Discover a new sense of identity and meaning with attention deficit hyperactivity disorder. Routledge.

Solden, S., & Frank, J. (2019). *Workbook for women with ADHD: A guide to emotional self-regulation.* New Harbinger Publications.

Solden, S. (2019). *Women with attention deficit disorder: Embrace your differences and transform your life.* Revised and updated edition. New Harbinger Publications.

Torgersen, T., Gjervan, B., Rasmussen, K., & Nordahl, H. M. (2018). *ADHD in women: A systematic review of prevalence, diagnosis, and treatment.* ADHD Attention Deficit and Hyperactivity Disorders, 10(5), 499–515. https://doi.org/10.1007/s12402-018-0265-9

Tuckman, A., & Severino, M. (2018). *More attention, less deficit: Success strategies for adults with ADHD.* Specialty Press.

Weiss, M., Murray, C., Wasdell, M., & Greenfield, B. (Eds.). (2019). *Women and ADHD: A clinical guide*. Routledge.

◆ ◆ ◆

Made in the USA
Monee, IL
08 November 2026

67383079R00156